7 Secrets Every Pregnant Woman Needs To Hear Before Giving Birth

The New Midwife's

R.O.A.D. To Birth™

Hypnobirth System

7 Secrets Every Pregnant Woman Needs To Hear Before Giving Birth

The New Midwife's R.O.A.D. To Birthᵀᴹ Hypnobirth System

First edition published 2022 by Nicole Schlögel

Essentiallybirth.com

About the author

Nicole is a mother, midwife (BSc), Hatha Yoga teacher, aromatherapist and educator. Nicole has been passionate about birth and holistic health her whole life. Working as a caseload midwife taught Nicole that pregnancy, birth and postpartum are interrelated and that holistic and nurturing care throughout this time forms the foundation for the journey of parenthood. This understanding led her to study with teachers all over the world, enriching her practice and experience. Her training as a Hatha Yoga teacher finally brought everything together and Nicole now runs the pregnancy, body work and birth preparation service Essentially Birth. She offers her services to a diverse group of clients face to face in Northern Ireland. Her online services can be accessed globally on **essentiallybirth.com**.

Download your bonus materials here:

https://www.essentiallybirth.com/ sevensecretsbonuspage

Dedication and Acknowledgements

This book is dedicated to my daughter Lena who was first to teach me about the practical side of pregnancy, birth and bodily autonomy. She also taught me how to be a mum, how to see the essence around which our bodies are assembled. She was with me even before she was fully embodied. It has been the greatest pleasure of my life to watch her grow and blossom into a young woman. She's the most perfect baby one could ever wish for.

Her father, my man Gerald, has been there for all of it, the good, the bad and the ugly. He too knows our daughter's spirit. Most of all he has been by my side through all my years of midwifery (only a midwife's companion can know what that means). Christmases on call, sports days, school drop offs and pickups, Sunday walks along the beach just the two of them because I was out supporting a mama. He made it special for Lena whenever he could and I am forever grateful.

I want to thank my parents for bringing me up wise enough to choose a good man and my mum and granny for teaching me the important stuff in life; letting my love flow into cooking, sewing, crocheting, knitting, baking and to look after my health.

And then there's you, the pregnant mamas, you have taught me to be humble, to know my place in this eternal circle of life. You have taught me what women can do and most of all you have shown me the R.O.A.D. To Birth. To every single family I have ever had the privilege to go alongside during this incredible time in your life - Thank YOU!

And thank you to midwives Evelyn, Kathy, Helen, Jean and Anne (the caseload team) for being the most amazing team to ever be part of. There's so much I could say about the years of being a caseload midwife among these women and about looking after pregnant mums and families the way we did but there truly are no words to do justice to how fulfilling an experience this was. Evelyn, thanks for being my 'other half' during all of it!

Finally, thank you to my amazing volunteer proofreaders. Jen, thanks for the thorough edit and all the hours you spent in the very early mornings and late evenings (I spied on you via modern technology). Mostly, thanks for encouraging me to knuckle down into the fine details and for your amazing feedback. Helen, thanks for giving me confidence in my R.O.A.D. To Birth system, for reading the whole thing a few times over and for being one of my most inspiring friends and mentors. Tara, thanks for being such an awesome fellow yogi, for allowing me into your space so generously and for putting a yogi's glasses on when proofreading my first draft. Thanks to Jodie, Paula and Séana for your feedback as pregnant mums. For reading through everything with such openness and for your honest feedback. Each of you has added value to this final version of the book.

Contents

Introduction

Hello and thank you for deciding to spend some time with me.

The fact that you have picked up a book about giving birth makes me think that you are either pregnant or planning to get pregnant soon. Either way, this is the book for you and if you are already expecting a little one, then I am extending my heartfelt congratulations to you. There really isn't a journey more rewarding than the path of motherhood.

In this book I will reveal to you seven secrets that every pregnant woman needs to hear before giving birth. I am telling you these because they reflect common misperceptions that I hear often when I talk to parents-to-be. They hold people back from following their instincts when it comes to making decisions about their pregnancies and the births of their babies and ultimately they generate fear. Learning about these seven secrets and then joining me on the R.O.A.D. To Birth will help you make decisions that are right for you and your baby from the start of your pregnancy. You'll look forward to giving birth without fear and on your terms.

Whether you decide to give birth swimming with dolphins or have a caesarean section in a state of the art operating theatre, this program will prepare you. You'll find out what questions to ask and how to ask for the things that are important to you.

In this book you will get the tools to figure out how you imagine the birth of your baby and you'll get the data you need to weigh up your choices.

If you have a birth partner, your birth partner and you will learn how to advocate for yourselves as a team. This will be particularly helpful if you don't choose to employ a doula or in settings where access for doulas or second birth partners is restricted.

Whether this is your first pregnancy or you are pregnant again, I am certain you will find value in these pages.

Why learn this - why not just leave it to the experts?

Many years ago as a student midwife I was taught that pregnancy is a 'normal event in a woman's life', have you read that anywhere yet? Are you feeling it?

My observation is that almost all women find this ordinary life event utterly extraordinary whether it's your first time or not. Pregnancy is a special state of being. Your body, mind and spirit are in a state of flux and expansion. You are growing a new human. You are going to give birth and you are going to nurture a child into adulthood. Pregnancy, as I see it, is as magical as it is mundane.

Meantime, once I was released to work as a fully fledged midwife in our modern maternity system, ready to support every woman and bump who came my way in whatever way they needed me to, I realised that the guidelines and protocols I am bound by don't lend themselves to treating pregnancy as a normal life event but rather a medical condition that needs to be closely monitored. You can see the dichotomy here, can't you? Midwives are taught that pregnancy is both a normal and a medical event, dangerous even. How are midwives meant to support you in your choices when there is such contradictory messaging in the very system we operate in? And then there's you all fluffy and pregnant and high on the extra oxytocin in your system. You don't even know yet all the choices you will be making by simply going along with routine care. How can I convey to you the implications of your decisions?

The answer is this:

Your care providers need you to be well informed.

First you need to decide what it is you are going after. Be it a natural birth, a caesarean or a homebirth, the same applies: You need to be informed to go after it and you will have a more positive experience being in the driver seat of your care.

What I have learned over the years of attending hundreds and hundreds of births is that no matter how the baby gets here, be it at a waterbirth or a planned caesarean birth, you are going through that transition. Each birth is transformational and carries with it potential for being a fundamentally positive and magically life affirming experience for you or it can bring trauma and suffering. Every time a baby is born, the mother is born too. Pregnancy and birth are the most meaningful rites of passage a woman can ever embark on. Every new baby does something new to you and a universal shift happens at each birth. Preparing for your baby's birth holistically can protect you from birth trauma, regardless of how your baby ends up getting here. Women who have an understanding of what is happening and why will find it easier to integrate their experience in a way that's meaningful for them.

The key lies above all in how well you prepare your body, mind and spirit for becoming a mother. Knowledge is power and the only variable that you can control is your own mindset. By doing that you will be able to line up the right support people around you.

Helping people like you be informed and able to take full responsibility for all your decisions as you walk through the gate to motherhood is what gets me out of bed every day. When you finish the last page of this book, it is my greatest desire that you will feel calm and excited at the thought of labour and birth.

Okay, but why should you listen to me?

Good question!

I am a mother myself. I have been pregnant, given birth to my girl and mothered her into adulthood. I have felt the elation but also the doubt and the fear that parenthood brings. But - and you might find that more reassuring still - I have also worked as an NHS midwife in the UK ever since I started on this path in 2005. So, apart from that time I got to give birth myself, I have seen hundreds and hundreds of births and I have supported thousands of women on parts of their pregnancy journeys. I have been a body worker and aromatherapist since before I ever became a midwife and I am a Hatha Yoga teacher. Knowing both a holistic and a medical framework to birth and birthwork and being on the yogic path gives me a unique angle to birth preparation.

I own the birth coaching company Essentially Birth and I offer my R.O.A.D. To Birth Hypnobirth Program online on zoom (and if you are local to me in Northern Ireland, you can join my face to face program and see me for body work sessions). I also teach a vegan pregnancy meal planning program called The Pregnant Vegan. My clients (not just the vegans) really love the meal plans and they enjoy adding extra plant protein sources and much more fruit and veg into their diets for a super healthy pregnancy and that's always a good thing, right? Send me an enquiry via https://www.essentiallybirth.com/contact-sevensecrets if you would like to know more about this. At this stage it would make sense to tell you that I have been enjoying a plant based lifestyle myself for more than 30 years and therefore I really only know how to cook plants.

I knew my calling to be a midwife early in life. I reckon I was about five years old when I decided that I would attend women in childbirth. My road to becoming a midwife was windy nevertheless. I first became an aromatherapist and worked as a bodyworker for a few years before I had my own daughter. My daughter's birth story gave me the resolve to finally become a midwife. I wish I could tell you it was because I wanted every mum to have a birth experience like mine but sadly that's not the case. My experience of giving birth was to leave me with scars and I couldn't talk about my daughter's birth without crying for many years.

The good news is that I have long healed and that ultimately my daughter's birth finally brought me on the journey to supporting families as a midwife. That's my vocation, it's my path.

Having had this perspective has meant that I will always be an advocate for unequivocally following the woman's choice once she has had a chance to look at all the different factors that form her big picture of pregnancy and birth. I love looking at data and the evidence that underpins midwifery and obstetric practice and then offering perspective on the guidelines and protocols presented to you when interventions are deemed necessary.

You'll read more about this later.

Meantime know this:

YOU - your body, your baby and your intuitive knowing - are as smart as any midwife or doctor - trust yourself to know what's best for you and your baby

What we will cover in this book

First I am going to let you in on seven facts about pregnancy and maternity care that will surprise you. They will debunk some commonly held beliefs and they will help you shed fear and recognise that you are the authority in your pregnancy and birth.

For instance, did you know that babies have 'cords around the neck' more often than you think and that it's not at all the drama and emergency people think it is?

Did you know that ultrasound scans to measure your baby are often inaccurate?

Or how about this one: For most women and babies homebirth is as safe as hospital birth, sometimes even safer!

I'll elaborate on those and four other misbeliefs that are floating around in the media and general public in the first chapter of the book.

This will set the scene nicely then for teaching you my simple R.O.A.D. To Birth Hypnobirth Program that I have developed over many years and that my clients love. You will learn a simple 15-30 minute daily routine that will transform your experience of pregnancy and leave you in excited anticipation of labour and birth.

Along your R.O.A.D. To Birth you will pick up why birth is a dynamic process between you and your baby. Birth is constant movement. You'll learn exactly how your body works in birth and how your baby moves with you and moulds into all of the available space inside your body in order to be born. It's totally magical!

Once your baby has travelled the distance, it's time to finally meet each other face to face. You'll learn how to best support your early postpartum time and how to start on your feeding and mothering journey.

Throughout this book as we explore aspects of pregnancy and birth decision making, I will refer to the bonus resources that you can access by following the links at the start and at the end of the book. You'll also find a reference list at the end of the book, you can use it to dive deeper into subjects if you want to.

Seven Secrets Every Pregnant Woman
Needs To Hear Before Giving Birth

Secret #1 'Going with the flow' is the worst idea ever!

I hear this a lot during first appointments, when I ask about a woman's preferences. I would looooveee a waterbirth/ caesarean/homebirth/ definitely an epidural' (doesn't matter what the answer is, really). Me:' Great! How are you gonna prepare for giving birth? Most common response: 'Oh, I'll just go with the flow and trust the experts.'

Is that you?

If it is, I am glad you picked up this book. Because, if you are choosing to give birth within the system you don't just need to know your own body and mind but also the system itself. Going with the flow without seeking information from the people who produce the current of that flow ultimately means going with the flow of the system. 'The flow' is very clearly defined by policy and guidelines for all kinds of scenarios according to your 'risk factors' some of which may not even be on your radar at all. For a positive birth experience you need to know what 'the flow' would be for you and how your provider is equipped to facilitate your flow if 'the flow' doesn't sound so good to you.

In my experience it's often first time parents who plan to go with the flow and it is often people who have had babies before and who applied this approach previously who are the most eager to set up a scenario where they are protected from 'the flow'.

If you are asking yourself what the heck I am talking about here, keep reading. By the time you have finished this book you'll have the tools to set yourself up for a positive birth whatever your choice might be. If your dream is a homebirth or a waterbirth, you'll learn where 'the flow' can have you drift away from this and if it's a planned caesarean birth, you'll know what parts of the usual caesarean birth flow you might want to tweak a little.

Your experience of birth has to be about you and your baby, not about policy and guidelines. And you can make that happen!

Secret #2: Homebirth is as safe as hospital birth for most women and babies

Did you know this?

I don't blame you if the answer is 'no'.

I can't tell you the amount of times I have heard someone say to me that homebirth is either dangerous, brave, selfish, unreasonable or even stupid. The public perception of homebirth is a lot of things but rarely have I heard someone say, sure, homebirth is the safest option for mama and baby.

But, counter to common belief, for many women homebirth is safer than hospital birth and no more dangerous for the baby.

When your next door neighbour tells you that homebirth is totally irresponsible, they are implying that the reason birth is generally safe these days is because it happens in hospitals and that is simply not true. Not according to a major systematic review published in the leading medical journal The Lancet in April 2020.

The finding of this very large systematic review and meta analysis of 14 studies from all over the world was that mothers and babies were just as safe at home as they were in hospital. Altogether, around 500 000 births were included in the meta analyses which makes this a very reliable finding. All the women in the studies were considered to be 'low risk' women, meaning that they were found to be at a low risk of birth complications. You'll learn more about what that means as you read on.

All these women were having their first babies and birth for little siblings is statistically safer again.

The interesting part is that women who gave birth at home were more likely to breastfeed their babies, less likely to have major tearing of their birth passage, less likely to bleed so heavily that a blood transfusion was required, less likely to have an emergency caesarean or instrumental birth and more likely to find their birth a positive experience. So arguably homebirth is safer overall because birth injury and birth trauma are important outcomes for a mother and breastfeeding your baby offers your baby health benefits that last a lifetime. The Lancet Study was done in two parts and both are in the references for the 'Choosing a place of birth' chapter. The two publications are easy to find online if you would like to look it up for yourself. If you would like a clickable link, sign up for the bonus materials and I'll send it to your inbox along with the other extra nuggets mentioned as you read on.

It is important to note that this data looks at women who plan to give birth at home attended by a midwife. There is currently no comparable statistical data available to evaluate the safety of the practice of planning to give birth at home unattended by a midwife, a practice commonly known as freebirthing. I have collated some information on the subject from the NHS and other sources in the evidence and decision making section of the book.

Secret #3: 'Cord around the neck' is rarely an emergency!

Just yesterday my client told me that almost every other person she talks to and discloses her plans to give birth at home to, responds by gasping 'But what if the baby has the cord around the neck?'

As a midwife I get asked the same thing frequently. There's just a whole lot of anxiety around this topic'. At this point I want to give a little shout-out to midwife and educator Dr Rachel Reed whose writings taught me what I should do about a babies' umbilical cord around the time of birth. The answer is surprisingly simple, in the overwhelming amount of births the answer is to do absolutely nothing!

Did you know that around 30% of babies have cords around the neck? We also have statistical evidence to suggest that babies with cords around the neck do just as well as babies who don't have cords around the neck!

This one seems to be really ingrained into society and people assume that the umbilical cord around a baby's neck will strangle the baby. In reality cords often loop around the baby's body and neck at birth and it's usually harmless. Around a third of babies come out with their umbilical cords worn as a necklace, this is because babies do a full circle around their own axis in order to be born. In other words your baby is like a little break dancer doing a head spin whilst still being tethered to the placenta via the umbilical cord. Hard to avoid getting wrapped up in it.

The umbilical cord is made for it though. It is wrapped in a special substance called Wharton's jelly, a fibrous type of gelatine that protects the blood vessels inside the cord from being compressed and therefore making sure your baby's blood supply is kept going even when the cord gets wrapped around the baby's body. Nature is magnificent and birth is safe.

So next time somebody tries to scare you by saying 'what if the baby's cord is around the neck?' (why people do that to a pregnant woman, i'll never know), you simply let them in on our secret #3 so they can relax and spread the word.

Secret #4: Ultrasound scans to measure your baby are more inaccurate than you might think (why there's no such thing as just a wee looksee)!

How accurate do you think an ultrasound scan is? Just take a guess? If the doctor tells you your baby is 4kg (8lb13oz) what size of a baby do you think we are talking about? Write down your best guess.

…..

So here's what the evidence says:

Most studies say that ultrasound scans to estimate your baby's current weight are up to 15% inaccurate. In other words, if you are told that your baby weighs 4kg (8lb 13oz), your baby can weigh between 3.4kg (7lb 5oz) and 4.6kg (10lb 4oz) (Dr Sara Wickham, 2021).

Wow! That's a big difference isn't it? But why is that an issue?

Well, say I told you your baby is 8lb 13oz, how would you feel about giving birth? Would you be more afraid than if I told you your baby is 7lb 5oz?

If you answered 'yes' to this question, your response matches that of many women I have spoken to over the years. And yet, the vast majority of 'big' babies arrive perfectly fine, in fact the biggest baby I have ever seen being born was born in the birthing pool. The baby was 11lb 3oz (5.1kg). None of us expected the baby to be this big, and so the baby *wasn't* big…until he was born. So, to an extent, your baby is as big as you think …until your baby is born.

The main issue with going for a scan in late pregnancy and having your baby's size estimated is that you are likely to be offered an induction of labour if the baby is 'big', despite the fact that we don't have any conclusive evidence to suggest any benefit in inducing labour for an estimated 'big' baby. You'll see later on in the book what an induction of labour entails and why it is best reserved for when it is really needed.

When it comes to your baby's size, I would encourage you to trust your own instinct. You'd be surprised how accurate you yourself can actually be, particularly if you have had a baby before. Is this baby bigger or smaller? But also a first time mama tends to know if the estimation is off the scale huge and totally not what she feels herself. Trust yourself, get a second opinion if you really doubt the estimation.

In any case, I always recommend that you know if you would want to have an induction of labour because of an estimated big size before you go for an ultrasound scan in late pregnancy. Obviously such decisions need to be made in the context of your health and pregnancy history and always in discussion with your own doctor or midwife, but knowing what you would do with the information gained at an ultrasound scan before you go is going to help you feel in control of your decisions.

To read a thorough evaluation of the evidence around induction of labour for all different scenarios, I highly recommend the book 'In Your Own Time' by Dr Sara Wickham.

Secret #5: The fiction of due dates

When are you due? Do you expect your baby to come on that day?

….

The medical model assumes that a normal pregnancy lasts 280 days (40 weeks) and that after that it gets dangerous for the baby. That means that your baby is thought to be due on the 280th day after your last period. Dr Franz Naegele described this rule in 1806 but unfortunately he didn't note if he meant the first or last day of your last period. That represents a variation of 3-8 days, the length of a monthly bleed.

The notion of a 'due date' is cemented into the very foundations of obstetric care in most parts of the industrialised world and as such it has been adapted and widely accepted by society. However, knowing how we came to determine when women are 'due' might help you make a more balanced decision about induction of labour at the end of your pregnancy.

Is there a standard gestation for all babies? Could individual babies and individual mamas decide their own timeline and what would happen if we stopped inducing labour because pregnancy is now deemed prolonged? I don't have the answers here but I know that these questions occupy a lot of pregnant women's minds.

We do know, though, that only about five percent of women give birth on their due dates, meaning that you have a 95% chance of not giving birth that day and by 41 weeks only 80% of women have gone into spontaneous labour (Corbett, et al., 2022).

This focus on the due date can cause a lot of stress and if you have ever been around a pregnant woman who is now considered 'overdue' you will know that the sense of anxiety and anticipation is palpable.

By the way, if you don't want to get bombarded with 'is the baby here yet' - messages, I highly recommend that you think carefully before you share your 'due date' with friends and family.

Just yesterday, one of my clients, who is expecting her third baby, told me that this time nobody knows her due date. She decided to give herself lots of extra time to go into labour without facing the angst of her loved ones. She just told everyone 'Baby should be here by the end of August'. She learned the hard way. She said 'Try going into labour when people are harassing you every day, amping up your anxiety by the hour.' Anxiety and the associated adrenaline is a definite barrier to starting your labour!

As you will learn as you continue reading, anxiety causes the release of the hormone adrenaline and adrenaline is NOT your friend before labour. Adrenaline competes with labour inducing hormones and can delay the onset and the progress of labour.

The modern obstetric paradigm and the associated NICE (2021) guidelines on induction of labour now recommend that all women be offered a conversation about an induction of labour at 7 days 'overdue, given that only 5 % of women go into labour at 40 weeks and 20% of women are still pregnant at 41 weeks, the likelihood of having an induction of labour offered to you in an otherwise 'normal' pregnancy based on your 'due date' is relatively high.

This is a complex subject and each individual must make their own decision in communication with their care providers.

Secret #6: You could have gestational diabetes in Belfast but not in London!

It's not the Yellowman sweets or the love of the Ulster Fry here in Northern Ireland, no, it's policy!

Some hospitals follow guidelines issued by the World Health Organisation, other hospitals follow guidelines issued by the National Institute for Health and Care Excellence (NICE) and some hospitals follow their own guidelines. Yes, true story!

Hospital policy is driven by resources and by cost. Basically, how we can achieve the best possible outcome at the lowest possible cost is what commonly decides which policies are implemented. So you could have gestational diabetes in Belfast but not in London and vice versa, depending on the policy implemented in the hospital you go to.

I am using the example of Gestational Diabetes (GDM) in order to point out that pregnancy care varies around the world and even nationally in the different hospitals. This also means that you will find different inductions of labour rates, different caesarean section rates, different water birth rates and different homebirth rates across providers. Knowing this is important because as you will see in our 'Overcoming Obstacles' chapter, the variations can be significant and doing your homework before you register with a certain provider is worthwhile.

While getting a diagnosis of diabetes in pregnancy will change how your pregnancy is monitored and increase your likelihood of interventions, there is limited evidence to suggest that routine screening improves your or your baby's health outcomes. On the other hand it is important to know that GDM if left uncontrolled can cause your baby significant problems. As always it is about striking the balance when it comes to decisions around screening tests. You could take a preventative approach and follow a whole food plant based diet which is associated with lower overall rates of GDM due to its high fibre content (Pistollato, et al, 2015).

If you would like to know more about Gestational Diabetes, I have linked some amazing resources in the bonus materials. You will also find a detailed exploration of the topic under the heading 'Are you at risk of developing diabetes in pregnancy' in the evidence and decision making section at the end of the book.

Secret #7: You can say 'no' (or 'not yet')!

Any intervention is always only offered to you, even if this is not explicitly pointed out at the time. Most people do not know that they can decline any aspect of their care.

You alone get to decide what happens to you, your body and your baby.

I am telling you this because there are women out there who have felt pressured into interventions. They didn't know that in the vast amount of situations, there is time to pause and assess the big picture, to consult with your partner, to tap into what your gut tells you, to connect with your baby. They went with the flow and the sad reality is that birth trauma is on the rise and affects an estimated 30 000 women per year in the UK and part of this is down to not feeling fully informed about their choices.

So, if you are not sure about something, ask. If you feel that things haven't been explained fully and that the conversation is one sided and only promotes the benefits of an intervention, it's okay to ask what the downsides are of going down the suggested route right now and what would happen if you didn't.

Ask for statistics so you can compare absolute risk in each scenario (you'll learn more about this as you read on). Ask for time to decide. Ask for a second opinion if need be.

I know that every mother has her baby's very best interest at heart, more so than anybody else.

That is why I trust you unequivocally when it comes to making decisions for you and your baby.

Let's get on the R.O.A.D. To Birth

These seven secrets reflect on some commonly held beliefs about birth that scare parents and also on the fact that how your maternity system approaches your pregnancy care is different from place to place.

How many of the seven secrets did you know about already? Is there any one in particular that shocked you?

How your maternity system approaches pregnancy shapes our beliefs about birth in society. It therefore shapes your own perceptions and those of your friends and family. As you read on, you'll see how your beliefs shape your experience and how your experience shapes your beliefs.

As you read on, you'll get the tools to have a good look at your internal landscape and you'll get to ditch the beliefs that don't hold true and the ones that don't serve you. You'll recognise fearful thoughts quickly and you'll have the tools to let them go. With a bit of practice many of my clients manage to do this on the spot as a thought comes up. So can you!

When I practise midwifery, I try my absolute best to put my own bias to one side, provide you with as much evidence as I can and fully trust you to make the decision. To me, this is the only way I can show up authentically for you in your time of pregnancy and birth. This is how I am showing up here in this book to help you make choices that are true to your values and beliefs.

A big part of your journey will be figuring out where your locus of trust sits. Would you rather go with the medical version of birth, or would you rather place your trust in yourself, your own body? This is deeply personal and there isn't a right or wrong answer. Both options offer advantages and also bring disadvantages.

My Hypnobirth program is based on my experience of facilitating thousands of antenatal appointments and talking with women about the strengths and limitations of each approach and how to find where you stand in it all so you can make truly informed choices. It is called the R.O.A.D. to Birth Hypnobirth System. As you go through this program , you'll learn how to confidently make decisions that are right for you and your baby and take responsibility for them. Taking this approach of self-responsibility will set you up for the rest of your parenting journey.

The New Midwife's R.O.A.D. to Birth™ Hypnobirth System

What's the R.O.A.D. To Birth Hypnobirth System?

The R.O.A.D. To Birth Hypnobirth System is my approach to hypnobirth.

Hypnobirth is most commonly known for the breathing techniques that you will practise through your pregnancy and then use at birth. Hypnobirth also uses visualisations and affirmations in order to prepare you for giving birth. What most people don't know is that deep breathing practices combined with visualisations and affirmations are all rooted in traditional Hatha Yoga and they can be applied to all areas of life, not just birth. So you can stay on this R.O.A.D. for as long as you like.

In order to visualise giving birth, you have to understand birth in the context of modern maternity care and decide what parts of it, if any, are for you. The R.O.A.D. To Birth Hypnobirth System provides you with a solid understanding of birth in all its forms.

By learning how your body works in pregnancy and birth you will be able to visualise yourself and your baby in labour. You'll be able to imagine how your baby moves through you in birth and how your body moves around your baby and releases your baby into your arms. Have you ever considered that your baby is an active participant in birth, that your baby experiences being born while you experience giving birth? The iconic western spiritual teacher and yogi Ram Dass refers to this as your baby 'taking birth' which I find an interesting concept to play with. You'll be invited to reflect on all of this on your R.O.A.D. To Birth.

To me this is the kind of stuff that life is made of and that's why I have developed this system. The great thing is that by learning all of these things and by learning how to tap into your body's ancient blueprint, your experience of pregnancy itself is also bound to be so much richer and more miraculous regardless of how your baby is born in the end. You'll make space for the possibility of all outcomes on your R.O.A.D. To Birth and you'll learn how to plan for a positive caesarean birth so that you are prepared for all possible ways a birth can go.

Birth is not the end product, it's a process, it's your and your baby's journey together.

During my years of being a midwife and speaking to countless parents during their pregnancies I saw patterns emerge. Women encounter similar roadblocks when it comes to preparing for birth. Those roadblocks can materialise in different ways, but ultimately they can be dismantled in the same way and put into four categories.

The R.O.A.D. acronym explained

R - Recognise and Release Fear

Fear is holding women back. If it isn't their own fear, it is the fear that is woven into society and into maternity care today.

O - Overcome Obstacles

Maternity care systems and the associated policies can pose many obstacles to an autonomous and self directed pregnancy and birth and sometimes the obstacles are in your own mindset.

A - Accept what you can't control

Sometimes your path will deviate from what you expected and you'll have to adjust. You'll also have to accept the practical implications of your choices be it inside the maternity care system or outside of it.

D. - Do the work

The day you give birth will be a day you remember forever. Prepare for it, research your options, learn about your body. Implement a daily breathing and visualisation practice into your routine.

So, in summary, the four steps on your R.O.A.D. To Birth are:

- Recognise and Release Fears

- Overcome obstacles

·　Accept what you can't control

·　Do The work

Together they give you a systematic approach to observing your own mindset and adjusting it for the best and most satisfying birth as you go along. You'll have the tools to let go of fears and to cope with whatever your pregnancy brings. You'll be able to distinguish between interventions that are based on real life and death situations and interventions that are purely routine and triggered by hospital protocol. Finally, you'll learn how you can implement little bits of practice into each day that will easily add up and have you ready to deal with the emotional and physical task of becoming a mother.

Some birth basics

Before you start on the mindset work in your program, we need to have a brief look at how the different ways of giving birth are described by your care providers and by society in general.

When you give birth naturally, this can be called:

- A Natural Birth

- A Normal Birth

- A Normal Vaginal Birth

- A Spontaneous Vaginal Birth

- A Physiological Birth

- A VBAC (vaginal birth after a caesarean section)

When I think of a natural birth or a physiological birth, I think of labour starting naturally, and you giving birth with no medical intervention at all. Examples: a homebirth, hypnobirthing, waterbirth, an unattended birth or freebirth, a physiological birth in a busy labour ward, a spontaneous vaginal birth in a birth centre...they could all be called natural birth.

Normal birth in the medical model of birth has now been reframed as spontaneous vaginal birth in order to use less value assigning language. The intention is not to imply that it is abnormal to have a caesarean section or an instrumental birth. The term spontaneous vaginal birth describes a variety of scenarios. It could describe a birth without any intervention, as described above, but it could also mean a vaginal birth after an induction of labour and including an epidural but without the use of forceps or a vacuum cup. To the medical model, a birth is a spontaneous vaginal birth as long as no instrument was used to deliver the baby vaginally.

A VBAC is any type of vaginal birth after a previous caesarean section and it could include all of the above. A VBAC could be a homebirth or it could be an instrumental birth. Sometimes women describe their VBACs in terms of how many caesarean sections they had before giving birth vaginally. For instance a woman who had two caesareans before might call it a VBA2C, a vaginal birth after two caesarean sections and so on. On that note, the more caesarean sections someone has had, the more difficult they will find it to find support for a vaginal birth. This is why I talk about obstacles and how to navigate those in R.O.A.D. To Birth.

You can have an instrumental birth (assisted birth)

Instrumental births are performed with either forceps or a ventouse (vacuum cup).

The assessment as to which instrument would be most appropriate to use is made by the doctor and it depends on how far your baby's head is in the pelvis. A discussion about how you feel about the possibility of an instrumental birth should be an option for you during your pregnancy. A common reason for an instrumental birth is that you have been in the birthing phase (often called the second stage of labour or the pushing stage) for a certain amount of time and the baby hasn't arrived yet or your baby is showing signs of distress. Instrumental births are overall more common when you have an induction of labour or an epidural but they can also be deemed necessary without any prior interventions - there's more info and different considerations about your choices in this later in the book.

You can have a caesarean birth

A caesarean birth is also an assisted birth. It can be called

· A caesarean section or c-section

· A C/S

· An abdominal birth

Caesarean births can be called elective (planned) or emergency C/S. This simply distinguishes between ones that are planned ahead of time and you never go into labour at all and caesareans that are performed at any stage in labour.

There are some situations where a planned C/S is truly inevitable for either mum or baby and in other cases, the suggestion of performing a planned C/S is triggered by protocol. As you saw in secret #5, protocol can vary between institutions and the evidence to support the intervention may not always be crystal clear. There's also times where you may feel you prefer a planned caesarean birth despite the fact that there are no factors that would suggest it is indicated. These are scenarios where a conversation with a trusted care provider is very important so that you can make a truly informed choice. You'll find more information on choices and on planning for a caesarean later in the book.

R - Recognise and Release Fears

There's a process to discovering how we think about things. Sometimes we are not aware of our thoughts and therefore we don't check if they are actually true. For instance, I only started on my path to midwifery in my early 30s because I grew up being told by my mum that I couldn't be a midwife because I would faint at the sight of blood. So every time I thought about how I would love to be a midwife I immediately thought, bummer, I can't be because I faint at the sight of blood. I never tested this thought, I never questioned if it was true or even my own thought. Spoiler alert: Not true!!!

I meet a lot of women who tell me that all the babies in their families are born by caesarean and therefore they'll probably have to have one too. I also hear 'I always have to have my waters broken' from mums who have had babies before. Is that true? Would the baby come if you were left to your own devices? Another one I hear a lot is 'I don't deal well with pain'. Again, is that really true?

In this chapter you will learn to question your thoughts but also, you'll learn to recognise feelings that trigger thoughts and how to manage those. So come on a little journey with me. You'll get to dream a birth and to really explore your mind's tendencies.

Do you know the song 'Your only friends are make belief' by the Bloodhound Gang? There's a catchy refrain it it:

'Your best friend is you, I'm my best friend too, I share the same views and hardly ever argue…'

It's a 90s song, so maybe you missed it. It doesn't have to offer any insights other than this refrain, in fact it's quite rude, so don't listen to it if you are easily offended. Forgive me, I rocked out to it in my 20s. I just thought it would be a good line to use to make the point that we tend to agree with ourselves and I didn't want to steal the credit.

Anyways, I think we tend to agree with our thoughts, particularly the ones that limit us and I am encouraging you to occasionally disagree with yourself. You don't have to argue with yourself per se, but I would like you to become aware of your limiting thoughts and ask yourself 'is this true', particularly if the thought makes you feel fear. For instance if you think: 'I won't cope with the pain' ask yourself if this is true.

To find out what you are thinking about birth in the first place, go ahead and do the following few exercises.

Dream a birth

This exercise is about helping you get clear on what you want for the birth of your baby and also about digging deep to figure out your beliefs about birth. You are going to need to find out where on the spectrum you find yourself between these two opposites:

'Birth is a bodily function and I am totally equipped for it, I hold ALL the resources I need, I am a birthing goddess'

OR

'Birth is a medical event and attempting to do it without doctors nearby is ruthless, selfish and irresponsible'

Ask yourself truthfully which statement is closest to your beliefs. Most people are somewhere in between. Where you sit will guide your choices in pregnancy and digging deeper will show you where your deeply held beliefs might be holding you back from going for the type of birth you really want.

Have you thought about giving birth yet?

How do you see it? Do you see yourself with your partner or husband? Who else is there? Do you see a doula there? If you are lucky to still have your mum in your life, is she there? Are you on your own?

Where are you? Are you at home? Which room are you in? Or are you in a hospital, perhaps your ideal birth happens in a hospital theatre, it could be a caesarean section. Can you imagine your surroundings?

Maybe you are super calm in a pool of water quietly moaning, oozing your baby into your own hands? Maybe you are howling and roaring for your baby's grand entrance. What's the lighting like? Is it dark, or are the lights on? Is there a round theatre light pointing at your belly? You might give birth by candle light. It could be daytime and there's light streaming through the window. Is it sunny or is it a beautifully grey drizzly day outside?

What's the temperature like? What does your body feel like? Are you dressed at all or are you naked feeling the air move against your skin. Maybe you are wearing your favourite T-shirt, the one you've worn hundreds of times before for comfort. Maybe you are wearing a bikini top in the birth pool or maybe it's a theatre gown.

How much do you move? Are you dancing and swaying? If so, is there music? What music is it? What else do you hear? Are there any beeping machines or the bub bub bub of a CTG machine? Maybe there's total silence in between your sounds. Maybe you hear your older children in the kitchen? Is there any sound at all?

Do you have a sense of time? How long will your labour be? Maybe you imagine different parts of it, snapshots. Do you plan to move from your home to a birth centre or hospital? Have you imagined a car journey or have you not thought about it in such detail? Maybe you will call someone to your birth. Can you see yourself making the call?

What about the very moment you meet your baby? Have you imagined that yet? Where are you looking at your baby from? Are you kneeling, looking down at your baby? Do you scoop your baby up right away or only after getting a good look first? What about if the baby is born into the water?

If you are imagining a Caesarean section, how do you see yourself walking into the hospital? Are you very nervous or totally calm? What weather is it outside? Is it dark? What are the sounds, will you pay attention to them? Who will come with you? Have you imagined yourself during the different stages of getting your anaesthetic, being wheeled into theatre and getting ready to meet your baby any moment. Who is with you there? Does your baby go straight to you for skin to skin?

Do you ever imagine what your baby might look like? Can you see your baby's face, the little fingers, your baby's toes? Does your baby have any hair? What colour is it?

What do you feel when your baby is born? Relief? Gratitude? Elation? Love? Connection? Surprise? Pride? Go there. Allow yourself to feel it.

Part of preparing for birth is to imagine it. Imagine it often and imagine your ideal scenario. If you could dream it into existence, what would it be? Feel free to change the script as you learn more about birth reading on.

How to do your dream birth exercise

This exercise is designed for you to find your dream birth scenario. It is to focus your thoughts. Most of us daydream about the future without even being aware of it. You might have a little flash of a thought whilst driving to the grocery store or just before going to sleep. Let's get those thoughts on paper and add to them.

Being specific about your destination will help you map out your R.O.A.D. To Birth. Where exactly is it you are going?

Without knowing this you'll have no goal and with no goal you'll do what many parents do - 'go with the flow' (remember secret #1?).

For now, let's get clear on your destination. Take at least 30 minutes of alone time. Maybe go to a beach, a forest or your favourite cafe. Go somewhere special and bring a notebook and pen with you. This could become your pregnancy journal for you to capture thoughts and feelings over the next few weeks until your baby is born. It could be an account to give to your baby when they get older.

Here is a listed version of the questions for you to lean to when writing about your dream birth. They are just to get you thinking. Please don't restrict yourself to answering those, there will quite likely be things you need to include here that I haven't thought about. As you read more and learn more about birth, you might want to add things.

· **Where will you be?**

· **Who will be there?**

· **Will labour start during the day or at night?**

· **Will you go into labour at all?**

· **How long will it take?**

· **Is there a care journey at some point? Do you need to travel?**

· **Or will someone travel with you?**

· **What's the lighting like?**

· **What sounds are you hearing?**

· **What sounds are you making?**

· **What smells are you smelling?**

· **What's the temperature like?**

· **Do you feel a breeze on your skin?**

· **If you are going to theatre, who's with you as you arrive and later in theatre?**

· **Are you in the water?**

- What position are you in when you give birth?

- Are you oozing the baby into your own hands or is someone receiving the baby? If you are planning a caesarean birth, would you like to receive your baby skin to skin, could you assist the caesarean birth?

- Can you imagine the moment when you hold your baby for the first time?

- What do you feel?

- What happens immediately after the birth? How do you interact with your baby? Do you feed the baby immediately?

- Have you thought about your baby's placenta? Can you imagine how it will be born? How long will you be waiting for it?

- Does your baby's cord get cut or are you leaving it intact? If it gets cut, who cuts it?

After the exercise, close your book and let it all sink in. Take a walk, connect with your baby and let your baby know the plan.

When you are ready, move on to the next chapter.

Evaluating your dream birth exercise

Now that you have done your dream birth exercise, ask yourself these questions:

Did you find it easy to imagine your baby's birth? How did you feel as you imagined it?

If it's an ecstatic, orgasmic water birth, do you believe yourself when you imagine it? If so, why? Are you finding yourself holding back? If that's the case, why?

Do you see flashes of a TV drama type birth where you have to be rescued by a knight in shining armour? Would you secretly like to be 'rescued'? Be curious about yourself. Check in with any thoughts that come up. Ask 'why?'

How you imagine your baby's birth is shaped by your experience of birth so far, the stories you have been exposed to throughout your life. Maybe you have given birth before and carry those memories good or bad. On the other hand, how you imagine birth will shape how you experience your pregnancy and your experience of giving birth to your baby. This is how the story of birth in our society is a perpetual circle. The good news is that you get to decide how you feel about giving birth. You can work at changing any negative emotions and replace them with excitement and anticipation.

At this stage I will say that, no matter how much preparation you do, occasional doubts and even some fear are normal, especially as you approach the end of your pregnancy or if you observe a bodily symptom that unsettles you momentarily. They are likely to pop up here and there in waves. We all have our ups and downs about upcoming important events and putting a new human on the planet is not only important, it is life changing for everyone involved. Those butterflies in your belly about giving birth are part of the process. The tools in this book are designed to help you deal with those moments as they arise, not to eradicate them completely.

On the other hand, having paralysing fear every time you think about birth and not being able to shake it, or not being able to think about anything else is likely something that you need to address beyond the scope of the practices here. If that's the case, please seek some extra coaching or counselling from an experienced practitioner.

List your fears

Before you read on, write down an initial list of any fears and niggly doubts you have become aware of at this stage

I am afraid of…
My worst fear is…
What if…

If you can complete any of these sentences, it's definitely on your mind and worth looking at. Keep the list at hand so you can get it later when you start working on fear release.

Understanding physiological birth and the effects of birth hormones

I see physiological birth as a baseline outcome, simply because that's what we would resort to stranded on a desert island. A Desert Island Birth so to speak. Also, in my experience, when asked at the beginning of their pregnancies, the majority of women would like to have a variation of a spontaneous vaginal birth (maybe with epidural). Very few women I meet would like a caesarean section from the outset but if you do, there's no judgement here whatsoever, I hope you still feel as amazed as I do at our ability to grow babies, give birth to them and then continue to nurture them into adults.

Birth on a purely physical level

In today's maternity systems we focus to educate you on the physical aspect of birth.

Birth is frequently described as unfolding in three stages and you'll be able to read more about how we have come to observe the process of labour and birth in this way in the next chapters and in the evidence and decision making section .

Let's just establish this for now:

Currently your baby is living inside your womb. Your womb is a muscle that is the size of a pear when you are not pregnant. Each month it lines with soft tissue in preparation to welcome a little fertilised seed. You have a monthly bleed if no seed implants into the lining. If you are in a heterosexual relationship and neither you or your partner have issues with fertility, you get pregnant if you have sex around the time you release one of your eggs from your ovaries and a sperm fertilises this egg. Some couples have assisted conceptions. Either way, the fertilised egg arrives in your womb space and nestles into the soft lining. It 'implants' and sometimes you experience some light bleeding around this time.

Your baby grows bigger and bigger until you are ready to give birth. Your womb has now grown immensely and it has formed a thick layer of muscle at the very top, the fundus of your womb. On the opposite side of the fundus is the cervix, the neck of your womb. It's the shape of a bottle neck and it is tightly closed and sealed with a plug of mucus.

For birth to unfold you have to dilate and your baby has to flex and rotate.

Once you go into labour, your womb makes contractions and those contractions pull the tissue up towards the fundus. For your baby to be born, your baby has to tuck in their little chin and rotate through your pelvis. As this happens your cervix dilates. The tissue of your cervix gets pulled over your baby's head and opens like a turtle neck jumper.

You have three bones in your pelvis, the two hip bones and your sacrum, attached to your sacrum is your little tailbone, the coccyx. Those bones can move a little bit making room for your baby to come through. At the same time your soft tissues in your birth canal stretch. Once the cervix is pulled over your baby's head all the way, you are 'fully dilated'. The stage from when labour starts to this point is called 'The First Stage of Labour'.

Your baby now slips deeper into the birth canal until you feel an urge to push. The time between fully dilated and having an urge to push is called transition.

Now your baby moves through the birth canal with your pushes or your breathing (or both) and eventually your baby will be visible on the outside. When the entire top of your baby's head, your baby's crown, can be seen at the vagina your baby is crowning. With the next few contractions your baby's head is born and then usually with the next contraction your baby's body is born (it sometimes takes more than one contraction for the body to fully release). The time between transition and your baby's birth is called the 'second stage of labour'.

There'll still be circulation between your baby and the placenta via the umbillical cord. Your baby's first breath is triggered by the stimulation of the cooler environment, by being touched and by your voice. Once your baby's lungs are taking over the job of giving your baby oxygen the baby's cord stops pulsing and goes white. Your baby's placenta is born when your womb does a final squeeze and releases it.

Join me on zoom for a visual demo of this during my R.O.A.D. To Birth Hypnobirth Zoom classes.

Desert Island Birth - our hormonal blueprint

Pregnancy and birth is a sophisticated process between you and your baby. Your hormones are the main players in pregnancy, birth and postpartum and for the longest time we had little understanding of how hormones interact and what part the baby's physiology plays in it all. We are starting to glimpse at this mystery. Thanks to people who have dedicated their life's work to research this topic, we know much more about the hormonal landscape of birth than even ten years ago.

There's a further reading section at the end of this book, be sure to take a look.

Early pregnancy on our desert island

Your journey to how your birth will unfold starts the moment you conceive. Your body gets ready for the task of nurturing and then birthing your little one from the very first moments of pregnancy. Let's get back to our desert island and transport ourselves into the mindset we would have there. We would not expect an ambulance to arrive, we wouldn't expect morphine or an epidural or any of the factors that now play into how we imagine birth today. If you think about it, our bodies are still the same bodies that our ancestors had, our bodies are old and wise but our minds and our lifestyles are modern. Let's for a moment imagine we were in a world as ancient as our bodies' design.

How would we notice we are pregnant? Did you 'know' before you took a test?

Did you have tender breasts, miss your period and maybe feel *different*? And then later in your pregnancy, did your belly get rounder just as you started to feel little flutters?

That's the cues we have always had to tell us we were expecting to welcome a new life.

By the time you feel those little flutters and movements from your baby, your baby's placenta has formed from the yolk sac that supported your baby when it was just a little embryo. This mysterious and miraculous organ, the placenta, forms an interface between you and your baby. You can supply your baby with all the nutrients, hormones and antibodies they need and dispose of your baby's carbon dioxide. All of this happens without your and your baby's blood streams ever mixing just where your baby's placenta attaches to the inside of your womb.

Your baby is in communication with you all the time and our environments influence our babies. What you eat, drink, the air you breathe, it all impacts your baby. Did you know that your baby develops a sense of taste and smell inside the womb? Your baby swallows the amniotic fluid and the fluid tastes of your food.

It is a little harder to take on board that our babies are also aware of our emotions. Emotions are ultimately chemical reactions in our bodies. The hormones and neurotransmitters related to our emotions are thought to cross the placenta making your baby aware of your emotional landscape. Please don't worry about this though if you are occasionally feeling sad or stressed. It's good for our children to learn that this is part of life and that you can self regulate during stressful situations. The deep breathing exercises in this book will help you with this.

Your baby will start to be able to hear by around 25 weeks and apart from your music, your conversations and the different voices of the people around you, your baby will also hear your heartbeat and the other sounds that your body makes. The swooshing of your blood, the gurgle of your belly and the sound of your breath. Your baby also starts to be able to feel touch. The sensation of being contained in your womb and the gentle rhythmical tightness that comes with Braxton Hicks sensations get your baby used to touch. Braxton Hicks are the practice contractions that initially go unnoticed but become more noticeable towards the end of your pregnancy. Do you find yourself placing your hands on your belly more often than usual? That's another way in which your baby experiences the sense of touch.

Whilst your baby is learning and growing inside your womb, your own body prepares for giving birth and mothering your young infant. Your ligaments soften because of the hormone relaxin. The joints in your pelvis are now softer to allow for the shift in your bones that takes place as the baby travels through. You can feel a little more achy in your hips as a result, be sure to move, stretch and get a pregnancy massage to help. Your breasts are starting to make milk because of the hormone prolactin, you might even leak a little colostrum here and there. At this stage your progesterone hormone remains high enough so labour doesn't start yet. Your belly grows and grows and in it your baby gets more and more mature.

Late pregnancy and the hormone of love

Expect a sense of 'being done' with pregnancy towards the end and often there's a level of anxiety, too. What's ahead? Will I really be able to give birth to a baby? How will I cope? Will the pain be bearable? Will the baby be okay? These are all normal doubts most women experience. As you get closer and closer to giving birth your rising oxytocin levels will help you replace that anxiety with more ease and calm and oxytocin also encourages bonding at the time of birth. Oxytocin is the hormone of love, calm and of labour. Oxytocin makes your womb contract to move your baby through the birth canal, bit by bit, little by little. This can take many hours or it can be a whirlwind of sensations and a quick birth. We can't know ahead of time, that's part of the miracle.

In the final days of pregnancy you make more oxytocin receptors and your baby is sending you a hormonal message via the placenta to say, 'it's almost time mama'. You make more of your hormonal birth cocktail consisting of oestrogen, oxytocin and prostaglandin and the neck of your womb, your cervix, softens and your mucus plug may release now. That mucous plug is called 'a show' and a show can happen a few times, not just once.

Your body keeps making more and more receptors for the oxytocin to bind to. Interestingly you don't just make oxytocin receptors in your womb but also in your breasts and in your central nervous system and this is what helps you deal with the sensations and the pain of birth. Your brain also becomes capable of making beta endorphins more easily than at any other time in your life. Beta endorphins are the body's natural pain relief chemicals, they act like opium on your awareness and there's a 'floaty and fluffy' feeling at the end of pregnancy.

You tend to find yourself seeking to pause and rest. You like privacy and feel like staying home with your loved ones close by. Those Braxton Hicks sensations start to change. Maybe there's a pattern to them now? You could have some more noticeable sensations throughout a whole night thinking that this is it, labour is starting, only for it to stop again in the morning. That's normal and it can happen a few nights in a row even.

You start thinking 'soon' and you keep your loved ones even closer. Often things really 'kick off' for real in the evening as it gets darker. Most spontaneous labours are at night and that is because in the dark your melatonin levels rise, you relax and that relaxation triggers more oxytocin and the surges really start to pick up then. You will recognise a definite pattern, surges ebb and flow and they get stronger.

Giving birth on our desert island

Let's assume we are still in this ancient world, as ancient as the blueprints of our bodies. How do we deal with the pain in the absence of modern day pain relief drugs? We wouldn't expect to have to outsource our coping strategy, we would rely on what our bodies are made to do.

I imagine we would respond by changing position often during the sensations and try to rest in between them. Our thinking brains would switch off and we would surrender to the rhythmical repetition of resting and moving and moving and resting. We would follow only our own instincts. Movement would not be prescribed, nobody would tell us to lie down, get onto our all fours, walk, lie on our sides or sway. We'd just follow our ancient design for birth. Any movement would be instinctual. Our body would make more of its own opiate cocktail. The more we would be able to surrender and relax, the more oxytocin we would release giving us more surges and allowing our babies to be moved a tiny nudge each time. Little by little we would yield the soft parts of our bodies. We might moan or we might howl our bodies into surrendering to the process.

This would keep going until our cervix was fully opened, we would be removed from this world. Our central nervous system and our perception of the outside world would be experienced through the veil of this sophisticated hormone cocktail, we would move in the rhythm of our labours, melting around our babies as our babies mould through us.

This state of being is still available to us in birth. We can still use our ancient blueprint to our advantage if we want to.

At the time of being fully opened your body releases adrenaline in order to take you out of this very removed and sedated state. On our desert island there would be no prescribed timeline for when this happens. Physiologically it happens when your cervix has fully opened and your baby can move through your birth canal. You are meant to be alert at this time so that you are able to protect your baby once the baby is born. This adrenaline release will make you feel fearful or even panicked. "I can't do it!' eyes wide open. Many women cry out, defeated 'I can't do this'. This is called 'transition' and once it starts to settle, a new resolve and sense of calm pours over you.

Often surges stop for a while now because of the adrenaline release. It can take a while for the oxytocin to become dominant again and for your surges to start again. 'Rest and be thankful' is what we call this time and it is a good idea to do this, to sip some water, maybe have a snack. Once you are refuelled and surges start again, your baby moves down further and moves onto your pelvic floor. Your surges become expulsive, your entire body works in unison, your womb contracts and your diaphragm and belly muscles assist with moving the baby down. Your sounds change and become more guttural, you are ready to give birth soon. This sensation is called the Foetal Ejection Reflex.

With a head down baby, this is when your baby really flexes their little head now so that their chin is on their little chest. This means that your baby's crown, the smallest possible part of the head, leads on the way out, gently, slowly continuing to stretch your soft tissues. The resistance from the pelvic floor helps your baby flex more and more and rotate their back forwards. Now the baby's head moves against your sacrum and your sacrum moves and creates a bulge in your low back, the Rhombus of Michaelis.

At this stage, women often instinctively move into an all fours position or a squat but not always. Instinctively we tend to favour a position that allows our sacrum (the bone just above your tailbone) to move freely. Standing, squatting or lying on our sides are all positions that allow this type of movement in the pelvis but there's no right or wrong position to give birth in. This is when to actually 'go with the flow', it's your flow this time.

Your baby is getting squeezed now. The little skull bones are moulding and moving on top of each other (don't worry they are made for that). The stress that the baby experiences at this stage releases adrenaline for them so that they can be alert for feeding once born.

It's a process in which you expand and your baby moulds through you. Your tissues stretch slowly, you may even expel some poo and pee to make use of all the available space in your body to allow the baby's passage into the world.

Your baby's head starts to crown and you may instinctively reach down to cradle the head, allowing the baby to ooze into your own hand. Follow your body, you may feel like moving your knees closer, that's the design of birth, go with it. It moves your sitz bones further apart for your baby's passage. Your soft tissues are going to sting and that might scare and startle you. It'll pass as your baby's head slips into your waiting hand.

Now you wait. You wait for the next surge and with it your baby's body is born. It'll take you a moment to realise that you have actually done it. This work of giving birth has challenged your physical, emotional and spiritual bodies in a new and unique way. You realign as a mother now. Once you have taken that in, you bring your attention to your baby. Your baby is taking a moment, too, being born and taking birth is a profound experience. You have literally travelled from one universe to another, the baby is now fully embodied on earth, claiming their space. The baby, too, needs to adjust. The adrenaline just before birth helps the baby to adapt to life outside the womb. The baby draws the first breath still attached to the placenta and you scoop your baby into your arms.

The first few moments on our desert island

You keep your baby skin to skin and the baby releases oxytocin which now starts to spread in the baby's blood stream replacing the adrenaline. You and your baby are primed for bonding at this stage due to the high levels of beta endorphins and oxytocin in your systems. The baby starts to root to your breast and the last bit of your baby's blood transfers from the placenta to your baby. It can take a few minutes for the cord to go white indicating that the circulation between the baby and the placenta has stopped and the baby's circulation is now independent from the placenta. Your baby's little hands are feeling for your nipple making it smell of amniotic fluid. Also, your nipples have a similar smell guiding your baby towards finally latching on. The baby's latch and sucking triggers a further release of oxytocin leading your womb to complete the birth by releasing your baby's placenta. This is a time when you will have the highest levels of oxytocin achievable in life.

This is an uncomplicated physiological birth according to our ancient design. As I said at the start of this chapter, I am not placing any value on it, we are merely using it as a blueprint to explore how external factors might influence it and how the modern obstetric paradigm might interfere with it.

Why fear is important in birth

You already know why fear is an issue in birth! If you have ever been afraid before, you'll know that fear produces a physical response and, intuitively, I think we all know that giving birth in fear would be very difficult if not impossible.

The feeling of fear serves a purpose in our lives. Fear can warn us of real dangers and in some situations fear is the only rational response in order to keep us safe. Just like we need to listen to the message pain gives us in our normal lives, fear can also serve a protective function.

Fear that is not based on reality can hold us back from living our life to its full potential. The what-ifs that are based on the worst possible scenarios are often not very likely to happen. It's the same in birth. Judging risk by the worst possible outcome is not helpful in balanced decision making. In today's society we are getting messaging that birth is dangerous from all around us. It's easy to be primed to fear the blueprint of birth.

In the next few pages we will explore the mind-body connection and how we can use our minds to regulate our bodies. We also learn how we can use our bodies to calm our minds, specifically our breath.

How fear works

Imagine that you are walking to your car at night in a dark car park. You are alone and you can't see very far. There are lots of opportunities for a potential assailant to hide behind the rows of cars you have to walk past to get to yours. Just thinking that someone is hiding somewhere in the dark ready to attack you, will increase your heart rate and make you breathe faster. Your shoulders are hunched, your eyes are scanning the dark for danger, you clench your fist ready to defend yourself. All this will happen automatically initiated by your parasympathetic nervous system. This response is called fight or flight. There's a purpose to this physical response, the extra breaths you take get more oxygen into your body and the increased heart rate pumps blood to your voluntary muscles more quickly so that they are at full capacity in case you decide to run. Meantime muscles that are not vital for the purpose of fighting or running away will momentarily get neglected and therefore they will not function efficiently.

Did you know that your womb is a muscle?

At the end of pregnancy it is the biggest single muscle in the human body. Quite impressive when we consider that it started out the size of a pear. In order to squeeze your baby out into the world, your womb will have to produce muscle contractions and, like any other muscle in your body, it'll need optimal blood supply to do so. You can guess where I am going with this can't you? In a state of fear, your parasympathetic nervous system gets you ready to either fight or run, not to give birth. The muscle contractions in your womb will slow down or stop when you are afraid. If labour hasn't started yet, it'll have to wait until you are out of danger.

We share this ability to stop labour in dangerous situations with other mammals who can easily find themselves being chased by a lion or a tiger. The modern human doesn't have nearly as many predators as wild mammals, nevertheless we are equipped with the same survival mechanisms and that means that, like all other mammals, we will be able to fully surrender to birth only when we feel safe.

The fight or flight response is triggered by the hormone adrenaline and we can conclude that adrenaline is not your friend in labour (at least up until the point of transition as you now know).

Unlike your uterus which is an involuntary muscle that is sensitive to the hormonal processes in your body, your skeletal muscles are under your conscious control. This means that you can decide to use them. Even though you might not usually be aware of the many decisions you make, you move through your day deciding to use your voluntary muscles. For instance me, just now, as I am typing these words, I am choosing to move my fingers across the keyboard. I can decide to either tense or relax my voluntary muscles in order to generate movement. The tense shoulders in our car park example demonstrate how your voluntary muscles also respond to fear. You tense them when you are afraid or in response to stress, you do it subconsciously.

Have you ever caught yourself as stiff as a board thinking of something that is stressing you out? Probably! Have you ever tried to consciously relax tense voluntary muscles? Do you find it easy to do?

The trust-release-bliss-cycle

So, we have established that just thinking of a possible threat releases adrenaline, increases your breathing and your heart rate and makes your muscles tense. The good news is that with a bit of practice you can reverse your fear response.

By simply deciding to slow down your breathing, you can regulate your heart rate. Once you are aware of your tight muscles, you can decide to relax them, making your body soft and subtle. This decision to relax becomes easier and easier the more you practise and by the time you give birth, you can choose to do this each time you are feeling the sensation of a labour contraction. Consciously softening your voluntary muscles makes it much easier for your womb to move your baby. Tense tummy and pelvic floor muscles directly work against the waves your womb makes to move your baby into your arms. Better still, consciously reversing the effects adrenaline has on your body will make your body stop releasing it and match the hormones to your actions. You'll release more oxytocin by running your body through its 'calm' program. You can actively assist the process of birth by learning to relax and once you relax and surrender to labour, your body gets flooded with that ancient cocktail of hormones that even dulls labour pain.

You enter what I like to call the Trust - Release - Bliss Cycle:

The more your brain is immersed in those hormones, the more relaxed you feel, the more relaxed you feel, the more labour hormones you release, the more labour hormones you release, the more labour progresses, the more labour progresses, the more your body and brain get flooded with the magic hormone cocktail, the more magic cocktail the more your mental state gets altered and the deeper you dive into a calm ocean of ever more labour waves bringing you to your baby, your baby to you. Your body has everything you need to get through labour and birth.

This doesn't mean that you never make a sound, doubt yourself, feel any pain at all or resist the process. It also doesn't mean that you have any guarantees about how your baby will be born, we never do. What it does mean, though, is that you can surrender to knowing that eventually every baby is born. You can also relax knowing that if you are reading this book in a place where you have access to medical care, you really have the best of both worlds. Birth is overall very safe, the journey is your own and the better you can get to know your innermost fears, the easier it'll be to deal with anything on your journey and surrender to birth.

The fear-tension-pain cycle

...the flip side of the Trust - Release - Bliss cycle.

When you are scared, you release adrenaline and we have already established that adrenaline is not your friend in birth. Adrenaline inhibits oxytocin production. Adrenaline is the hormone that makes you alert and ready to run. It produces tension. Tense muscles in themselves are painful and tense tummy and pelvic floor muscles can hold your baby in the current position making it much more difficult for your womb to move your baby to you. Adrenaline may be present because of your own subconscious fears or because of a fear inducing environment (hello sunglasses, and ear muffs to dull the bright lights and beeping machines in the busy hospital admission units). If adrenaline is dominant over the magical hormones, the beta endorphins and oxytocin you'll not get to the blissed out state of consciousness and therefore you'll experience more pain.

The British obstetrician Grantly Dick-Read described this as the 'Fear - Tension - Pain Cycle' in his book 'Childbirth Without Fear' which was first published in the 1920s. Assuming that pain out of context is scary, we can agree that the cycle could be this: The more fear, the more tension, the more pain, the more fear...

It's a vicious circle that you can break!

If you have identified that you think that birth is dangerous, then breaking the cycle starts with getting to the bottom of why you think that. If you are afraid of particular scenarios, it's time to get out your list of fears so you can find out as much as you can about them.

As a midwife of seventeen years I know that any scenario you could possibly imagine is either not actually as dangerous as you might think (see secret #3) or so incredibly rare that a simple mindset shift can help you overcome this fear.

Working on your fears now means that you can go into labour with confidence and trust in yourself and in your baby. You can get riding the Trust - Release - Bliss - Cycle.

Why fear is important in any type of assisted birth

Your baby's birth is going to be etched in your memory regardless of how your baby gets here. You will want to associate it with a positive experience. Working early on releasing any fears you may hold of a caesarean birth or an instrumental birth will open you up for the potential of experiencing ANY type of birth as positive.

Being free from fear also means that you will have the confidence to ask your questions openly and you are open to any information you receive. This is likely going to reduce your fear further.

If you choose a planned caesarean birth or one is absolutely necessary for your or your baby's survival (really only the case in very rare situations), then the techniques in this program will help you work around your specific fears.

You'll be able to:

·   Ask for a gentle caesarean and make your priorities and wishes known

·   Sleep better the night before

·   Stay calm when you are getting your anaesthetic with the obstetric doctor and nurse

·   Stay calm during the surgery if you are opting to stay awake

·   Be in a positive state of mind when you meet your baby

Instrumental births and emergency caesareans are less likely to happen in labour if you have started out in a homebirth or birth centre scenario using your techniques. If either one of those arise, your techniques and mindset can keep you calm and focused. In a scenario like that, this book will help your birth partner to draw your providers' attention to your birth plan and wishes.

I once looked after a woman in labour who was using breathing and mindset techniques to prepare for giving birth. She had been in labour and working at breathing her baby down (and later trying to push her baby out) for a long time. The doctors suggested a caesarean birth and she agreed.

When talking to her about pain relief the doctor said, 'You've got a well working epidural, all we need to do is top it up for your caesarean' to which she responded, no I don't have an epidural, I am using my breathing techniques.

The doctor turned to me and said, 'Does she not have an epidural?' and I said, 'no she doesn't'. The doctor now doubted her and me enough to double check 'are you sure?'. I laughed, 'I think she'd know if she did'. Even in the deepest throes of labour, my client had to giggle, too.

The woman continued her breathing techniques and remained so focused and calm throughout getting a spinal anaesthetic and through the caesarean birth of her baby. She later told me that she absolutely loved her experience of giving birth. She was.so.proud!!!

The ripples of positive birth (or why I get out of bed every morning)

I have many stories of women who addressed their fear in pregnancy and as result had a positive birth, but there's one message I got out of the blue one night that just hits the nail on the head when it comes to expressing how one positive story has the power to impact on generations of women.

I got this message from a woman who found me ten years after she had given birth. This message is everything to me because it shows how a beautiful birth story can impact on how a young girl embodies her place on earth. Imagine knowing that your birth brought your parents nothing but joy. I have no doubt that her birth story will shape this young girl's belief in her own ability to give birth to her future children, too.

'Hi Nicole. You looked after us ten years ago when I had my little girl. My husband and I arrived in the unit in the morning, on the lower slopes of our fourth labour. You supported us throughout the day, gave us our space, let us do our partner yoga until our baby arrived. So, I'm contacting you because we were talking at dinner this evening about her birth story and a wave of gratitude for you came over me. Your respectful assistance at her birth allows us now to share that experience with her, and I could see the delight in her face when she learned what a positive experience we had when she came into the world. That's a precious gift to be able to share with her and I just wanted to say you made that possible. Thank you. R.'

Imagine how much healing there can be if we claim our innate ability to give birth without conforming to protocols and hospital systems when it feels wrong to do so. This woman didn't want to have any interventions and she had a plan of how she was going to give birth. All I did was keep her birthing space free from distractions and observe her and her baby calmly and discretely. You can set yourself up for a birth like this too. You will get the tools in this book to make decisions that are right for you and you will learn how to communicate your decisions to your care providers. Your birth partner will know how to step in and allow you to stay in the zone if your providers need to find out your preference if a new situation arises.

I know that not all of us get that type of birth story and (like me) you may already have a child who doesn't have this type of story either. If that is the case and if my suggestion that positive birth stories can have lasting impacts on generations to come makes you feel uncomfortable, this is my invitation for you to explore your emotions with curiosity and love.

I know for certain that it is possible to heal from a traumatic birth experience. You can integrate our own birth story or the story of how any of your children were born and make them part of your healing journey on your R.O.A.D. To Birth.

How your own birth story can be in your way

I believe that we remember our own births even if we were never told the story. We were there and even though we usually don't have any conscious memories of it, it's written in our subconscious.

Did you grow up being told how you were born?

As you saw from R.'s story, our birth experiences span multiple generations and one negative experience can change the perception of an entire future family lineage as much as a positive story can.

I have a friend who grew up knowing that her own birth was traumatic for her mother and for her father. She was born in a remote village and as a child she was told all the details of the rare complication her mother experienced shortly after she was born. My friend's father had to go fetch some life saving equipment in his own car driving to the nearest city hospital and return with the equipment. He experienced immense anxiety during this lengthy round trip, fearing for his wife's life.

This type of scenario where a family member has to run such an errand luckily is far-fetched for most women in the UK today, however, growing up with this story meant that my friend feared birth. To her, birth was inherently dangerous and painful. In her mind women needed to be in a hospital surrounded by machines, doctors and equipment in case they needed saving. My friend spent her entire pregnancy afraid of giving birth. Of course my friend didn't experience the same emergency her mother had experienced but her labour and the birth of her daughter were difficult and traumatic.

I have seen many examples of trauma stemming from the expectation that labour is painful and dangerous and from expecting the solutions to come from the medical system and unfortunately the system can't do that. Midwives and doctors don't have all the answers and it is impossible to outsource the transition to parenthood fully. I find that fearing birth often runs in families. I see it when a woman brings her mother to the birth as a birth partner. If that granny-to-be believes that birth is inherently dangerous I usually find myself midwifing two generations in one birth room.

How to work on releasing your fears

Now that you know why fear holds you back when it comes to labour and birth let's get working on how you can start to release it. At this stage I want to reiterate that it is totally normal to feel fear here and there in pregnancy. Some of your fears may even pop up in labour again and that's okay. Having a baby is a big deal. How am I going to cope in labour, how will becoming a mother (again) change me…these are all totally normal thoughts and there's nothing wrong with you if they keep popping up. The techniques we are exploring here may help you to totally forget about a fear but if a fear seems stubborn and keeps popping up in your mind, then you'll have practised how you can consciously facilitate your body to reverse the physical effects of this fear.

Here are my go to techniques for fear release:

- Fact checking your specific fears

- Letting Go Technique

- Deep Breathing

- Meditation

- Affirmations

- Help From Outside

Let's check them out.

Before you move on, it will be helpful to have the list of fears and doubts you made earlier.

Fact checking your specific fears

Judging risk by the worst possible outcome generates a lot of unnecessary fear. There are countless examples of alleviating fear by simply noting how unlikely a situation is to arise. You also may have your facts completely wrong and your fear isn't even a thing that ever happens. This is where fact checking comes in.

In order to fact check your fears, you will need to name them. You will need to be specific about what they are. If you haven't already made a list when you evaluated your Dream Birth Exercise, do it now.

What are your fears? Go ahead and make a list.

I am afraid of ...

1. ....

2. ....

3. ...

....

Keep this list and go on a fact checking mission.

Can you gather some statistics? How likely is the thing to happen to you or your baby?

Is there anything you can do to make it less likely? The evidence and decision making section in this book supplies you with a rich resource and you might find some of your fears addressed there.

Is the fear even rational? I mean you could have a fear of a tiger chasing you in labour but that's an unlikely scenario where I am. On the flip side, if you are planning to put your birth pool up on the second floor in your apartment and you have a niggling doubt about whether your ceiling will support the weight of the water, do check in with that. It's entirely within the realm of possibility to crash into your downstairs neighbours' living room and therefore that's a rational fear.

Later you will learn how to turn your fears into positive affirmations that can help you deal with rational and irrational fears as well (no, I know, simply affirming 'My Pool Will Not Come Through The Ceiling' won't work but they can be magic otherwise!).

The letting go technique

The letting go process is described in detail in David Hawkins' book 'Letting Go, The Pathway Of Surrender'.

It's incredibly simple and yet very powerful. It's also rooted in yoga which makes me love it even more! You can almost instantly release a fearful thought and even regulate any physical response you might be having about the thought. For instance people who are prone to panic attacks use this technique to avoid an episode.

Our feelings are like waves and just like waves they can overpower us.

Have you ever played in the sea and jumped into waves before?

Do you know how differently you can experience a wave, depending on how you approach it? You can get knocked over, or you can glide through.

I remember sitting at a shore as a little girl. My cousins were meant to keep an eye on me but they decided to wander off with their friends instead. They figured they would just dig a stick into the sand for me to hold on to when the waves came. I was under strict instructions from the adults not to go into the water, not without my mum or dad! The idea of the stick seemed plausible to me at four years of age and so I stayed sitting at the shore, feeling grown up all alone by the water holding onto my stick.

It was nice for a while, I enjoyed the water washing over my little legs as I held on to my stick. Then a big wave came totally out of the blue and it washed me right into the water. I was fighting, flapping my arms, head under the water, gasping for air (still holding the stick in my hand somewhat surprised at how it had washed into the water with me). I was being spun around in the wave and I had no control. Luckily one of the adults had seen it all and came fishing me out of the water.

I have since learned that fighting a wave is pointless, you get swirled and bashed around. You don't have any control over where you get washed up again and what state you'll be in. And yet you could experience the same wave with absolute control.

Imagine seeing a wave roll in recognising that it could knock you over and instead of letting it crush and churn all over you, you decide to glide through it. You just dive right into the water below the crest and you glide. Same wave and yet an absolutely different experience.

This is how it goes with feelings.

Feelings are created through experiences and then memorised. A situation happens and it triggers an emotional charge, we form a thought about the situation and make a memory.

Going forward, that same thought will recall the memory and we experience the same emotional charge or feeling that we had when we first experienced the situation. The longer we live, the more experiences we gather and the more emotional responses can be conjured up by thought alone. Our emotional response becomes a habit.

You can relate to this, right?

If I ask you to recall a happy situation and explore every aspect of that memory, you'll respond by smiling and by lifting your emotional charge, your vibration, to the level it was during the happy event. And that works vice versa too. You can recall something sad and lower your vibrational state.

Sometimes there doesn't even have to be a prior experience for you to feel a certain way about a thought. For example, every time I walk to my car after having attended a birth in the middle of the night, I am scared stiff and yet I have never been attacked and hopefully I never will be. Yes, that car park scenario I described earlier was me walking across the hospital car park on many occasions. Same thoughts and fear program every time!

Emotions are chemical responses in our bodies and over time we get used to a certain level of emotions. We feel most comfortable in a familiar emotional state. You could say we are addicted to the chemical response certain emotions give us and therefore we tend to think the thoughts that trigger the emotion to produce the chemicals regularly. Most of the thoughts you are thinking today are thoughts you thought yesterday, in fact 95% of the 60000 thoughts we think on an average day are not new. It's easy to get into a funk thinking the same fearful thoughts every time you think about giving birth too.

Here's how we can deal with our feelings:

- We can suppress them by consciously pushing them into our bodies. Have you ever felt like voicing a certain opinion but then decided not to in order to fit in with the crowd. Suppressing our feelings usually happens when we want to fit into socially acceptable norms.

- We can repress our feelings. That's when we subconsciously push them to the side and carry them deep in our bodies. This usually happens after a trauma response. You may not even have a conscious memory of the event, memories can sometimes pop up in flashes.

- We can express them by acting them out in the situation. That way we address them in a timely fashion but it's not always good. People can be short fused or very emotional when they freely express their feelings all the time. You can observe this in young children who are learning to deal with their emotions.

- We can escape them and distract ourselves. Netflix anyone? Other ways of distraction are alcohol, drugs and overworking.

It's important to find a balance. None of us are always on top of all of our emotions. It's a constant journey and we constantly process new experiences. The goal is to become resilient and to teach our children to be resilient, too. Being able to take ownership of our emotions is a huge step towards self-responsibility. Understanding that nobody can 'make us feel' anything and that our emotional responses really are the only thing we can control in any given situation - and then holding ourselves true to that - is hard work but immensely liberating. Good emotional housekeeping means that you can stay clear from slipping into victim mode. It means that you become a neutral observer of situations rather than judging yourself or others for their part in it. By knowing your feelings and dealing with them as they arise, you can foster an inherent sense of self responsibility and ultimately you can enjoy freedom from guilt, resentment and fear.

Here's how to let go according to David Hawkins:

1. Become aware of the feeling and name it.

2. Become the observer and separate your identity from the feeling.

3. Experience the feeling without judgement, allow yourself to just *be* with the feeling.

4. Accept the feeling so that you can move through it.

That's it, done!

Practically, let me tell you what this might look like.

Back to me walking to the car at night. I know that it is highly unlikely that something will happen to me based on all my previous experiences and based on the fact that I am not aware of anyone ever having been hurt at this car park. I know that the chances of the worst possible outcome are low and my plan B is to just run for it.

Yet, as soon as I step out of the birth centre knowing I have to walk past hedges and trees towards a dimly lit car park I have the familiar emotion/ thought process going on in my mind and immediately I can feel my body's response. At this stage I have a choice. I can wait til it's no longer dark and let my fear paralyse me or I can walk to my car despite the fear.

Here's what I do to get on top of it:

I think, oh, here we go, Nicole's afraid of getting attacked, that's okay, that's just what she has to do (I am naming my fear and I become the observer without judging myself, I just *feel* the fear). I also know that this feeling does not define me. I am not this fear, my essence is separate from the fear, I am not my thoughts, I am not even my body. My consciousness is not afraid. Over time and with regular deep breathing and meditation practice in other contexts I have gotten good at becoming the observer of myself rather than *be* my body if that makes sense. Just that shift and the process of acknowledging my fear without judgement allows me to move through it smoothly and quickly as I walk towards my car. Before I know it I have turned the key in the ignition. Boom, job done!!!

This business of not judging yourself is the important part. I could easily go off on a thought tangent along the lines of: 'Arrrgghhhh I feel this way every time, I'm so stupid. Can't even walk across to my car without drama.' My inner dialogue could then get me more and more convinced about how weak and useless I am and about how I just can't do anything much by myself.

Judging our feelings can distract us from actually dealing with them. We can get carried away and still resent ourselves and others. I could make a list in my mind: the broken street lights, the fact that there's no security around the hospital, the fact that I always get called out at night…you get my drift.

In the context of a birth related fear it is just as simple. For instance the thought of 'I am not good with pain, I'll be a mess in labour' might pop up every time you think of giving birth.

So you just take a step back and observe your feeling. Say to yourself 'Ah, there's Sophie, she's afraid of the pain, that's okay.' Just allow yourself to feel the fear instead of fighting it or expecting that you should feel a different way. Move through it and move on. This can literally happen in seconds and it'll save you a lot of dwelling in fear.

Sounds simple and it really is! Try it out.

The sacred act of breathing

Our breath is life giving, life sustaining and we can make it life changing!

Breathing initiates our life outside the womb, it's our decision to breathe that gives us life. Our first breath marks our first step towards becoming physically independent from our mothers' bodies and our continued breathing is sustained by loving nurture, first from our parents and then we move on to nurture ourselves.

Tapping into the breath as a thread to the mystery of life and as a tool for self discovery and self regulation has been one of the most precious gifts in my life and I want to share it with you. The breathing techniques in the next few chapters can be some easy exercises and they can simply provide one of the instruments in your labour tool kit and that's perfect. The beauty is that they can be so much more. They can lead you on a spiritual path and to glimpsing more and more of the universal design and your place in it. And if that's not for you, that's totally fine, too. I am still sure you will find them useful beyond labour and birth because they have many practical applications for any situation that requires you to stay calm and collected.

What deepening your breath does for you

We have already established that fear can make you breathe faster and that the simple act of deepening your breath and slowing it down can reduce the physical effects of fear. It's just like the physical act of smiling can lift a gloomy mood. The mind follows the body, the body follows the mind.

Most of us are not aware of our breathing throughout the day, it simply happens. If we are very stressed our breath is generally shallow. Consciously deepening your breath and drawing it down to your diaphragm will relax you but it will also move the diaphragm muscle and therefore it exercises your pelvic floor which is directly opposite the umbrella shaped diaphragm muscle under your ribcage.

I personally learned to direct my breath via the practice of pranayama. Pranayama is one of the eight limbs of yoga and along with the seven other lifestyle practices taught in traditional Hatha Yoga, pranayama offers a path to connectedness and health. There are many different pranayama exercises you can move on to once you have learned the full yogic breath, sometimes referred to as sectional breathing or three part breathing.

Full yogic breath exercise

Traditionally the full yogic breath is done by breathing in through the nose and out through the nose. In pregnancy you might want to practise breathing in through the nose and out through pursed lips because that way you are more likely to keep the lips loose. Keeping your lips loose automatically helps you release and relax your pelvic floor in labour

The following exercise teaches you the full yogic breath in three stages. I would suggest that you practise each stage in isolation for a few days and then move on to the complete breath.

If you haven't left much time before your baby is 'due', go ahead and progress more quickly. I suggest that you spend ten minutes per day on deep breathing practice. You can do this as part of a yoga practice or just before bed time or in bed.

Breathing into the lower lobes = abdominal breathing or diaphragmatic breathing

- Lie on your yoga mat with legs bent, feet flat on the floor

- Lengthen your lower back by stretching the sacrum forward

- If you are past 25 weeks or you find lying on your back difficult, you can lie on your side with a pillow between your knees, sit on a chair or on your yoga mat in the easy cross leg position (Sukhasana) If you lie on your side, choose the side you prefer, for comfort.

- Let your shoulders ease back and down into the floor

- Lengthen through the back of the neck and relax your face muscles, tongue and mouth

- Place one or both hands onto your abdomen and begin to notice any movement there as you breathe

- After a few breaths, try to exaggerate this movement so that the tummy rises up a little more with each breath

- On each out breath let the tummy relax back towards the spine

- The lower abdomen below the belly button should not balloon out with this exercise

- Practise this for a few minutes

This increases blood and prana (life energy) to the lower belly, your womb and your baby, your pelvis, legs and feet. It also aids digestion and can help with constipation. It's useful in managing anxiety and panic attacks and is suitable for everyone.

Breathing into the middle lobes = intercostal breathing or ribcage breathing

- Stay in the same position and now cup your hands around your ribs

- Notice if there is any expansion of the chest when you breathe.

- Exaggerate this movement by pushing the ribs sideways as you inhale and allowing the ribcage to relax and narrow as you breathe out.

- You should feel expansion all around the middle of the body – practise for a few breaths

This breath helps to increase lung capacity.

Breathing into the upper lobes = clavicular breathing or upper chest breathing

- Now move your hands up around your upper chest, your collarbones

- There is a lot less movement here but you should experience some

- Direct breath to this area and try to feel that the breath also flows to the upper part of the shoulders and back – continue for a few breaths

The complete Breath

The complete breath is best practised in a seated position, so either on a chair or in easy cross leg on your yoga mat.

- Initially observe your breath and become aware of the ebb and flow of it – allow some time for the breath to establish

- Now breathe into the abdomen, continue the inhalation into the ribcage and then into the upper lobes of your lungs. Exhale a long slow breath and repeat this two more times.

- Rest and observe your breath in the here and now, no straining

- Try to slow down your out breath, you will learn how to do this more and more over time

- Counting on the inhale helps to learn the full yogic breath.

- Traditionally the full yogic breath is done to a count of two into the abdomen, two into the ribcage, two into the upper chest (total of six), and the outbreath is lengthened to 8 or 10, however you might find that difficult to do with your late pregnancy bump, so we modify it for late pregnancy and labour.

This practice lowers stress levels, strengthens the immune system and gives you increased energy. This technique is useful in early labour and in established labour. Doing three to four breath cycles will get you through each contraction (or surge). This type of breathing is often referred to as 'up-breathing'.

The complete yogic breath as labour breath:

This is sometimes called 'up breathing' because in labour, the muscles of your womb draw up a little more with each surge in order to let the baby slip down into the birth canal.

With the labour breath you breathe in through the nose and out through pursed lips, cheeks relaxed, face relaxed. You also introduce a count 4/8, breathing in for four and out for eight. If your baby bump makes 4/8 breath difficult, go for a 3/6 count. The important thing is lengthening the outbreath in relation to the inbreath, that's what calms the central nervous system. Counting puts your focus away from the sensation itself and to your breath.

Each breath cycle takes you around 12-15 seconds, assuming that a surge from the first niggle to crest, to rolling out fully takes 45 - 60 seconds, four labour breaths in a row will definitely cover you. So throughout the day, when you do your day to day stuff, just do some labour breaths, too. Each time you fold the laundry, cook your dinner, empty the dishwasher, ride the car or walk to work go ahead and practise four sets of your breath.

You can add your visualisations to this breath, for instance, imagine that your body is made of a beautiful warm malleable wax that moulds and melts away a little more with each labour contraction as your baby moves through you.

The birthing breath

The birthing breath is for when you start to feel your sensations change. You will feel some pressure on your back passage and you might feel an irresistible urge to push.Now instead of lifting up to move the cervix over the baby's head, your womb actually moves downwards to move your baby down. Remember that even though we are referring to the birthing breath as breathing your baby down, it is not wrong to push along with your body as long as this happens spontaneously and is not directed pushing with breath holding. Some women release their babies into the world without pushing and others do it with pushing spontaneously, the breath you use at this stage remains the same.

It's an active variation of the labour breath. You breathe in and on the outbreath you now blow the air out through pursed lips again but this time you imagine that you are blowing out a candle or you think of blowing at a feather trying to make it float across the room. No need to count, just breathe in and really blow all the air out of your lungs. If you have a wee go at this now, you will feel your diaphragm muscle moving down and your pelvic floor releasing. This way your accessory muscles can assist your womb in moving your baby to you. Start practising at around 36 weeks and do it every time you do a poo. That way you learn to release your pelvic floor and you may even find that you are straining less (particularly helpful if you have haemorrhoids).

Planting seeds for a joyous birth using affirmations

Positive affirmations are helpful in reminding you that you can and will give birth to your baby. They are also helpful in letting go of fears. A traditional yoga practice includes a positive affirmation at the start of your practice. In yoga this is called a sankalpa. A sankalpa is a vow to yourself, a seed you plant in your mind in order to nurture it into existence. There are many ideas for positive affirmations around to help you in labour and birth and I will give you some of my ideas as well. Generally, starting your affirmations with 'I am' is the most powerful way of self suggestion but you can also affirm what you choose to believe about birth or your baby for instance.

You can write out your affirmation onto some nice paper and pin them up around your house for you to see every day. Say them out loud, whisper them to yourself or just think them when you see them. Pin them up in your birth room to remind you of your affirmations and resolutions when you are in labour.

For affirmations to be relevant to you, I invite you to go and get your list of fears.

Now turn each fear into its direct opposite.

For instance if you wrote 'I am afraid that I'll need a caesarean section'', you can rephrase it into something like 'I am powerful and I capable of giving birth with ease', you can also affirm this: 'I am confident that the birth of my baby will be blissful and joyous in any circumstance". If you wrote 'I am afraid I won't cope with the pain', go for something like 'I make my own bliss hormones and pain relief' or 'All I need in labour is available to me at any time. I am strong'. This is personal to you.

Turning your fears into their direct opposites and affirming these positive opposites often will help your subconscious mind be reprogrammed.

Take a moment to write down your personal affirmations and place them where you can see them, for instance the bathroom mirror, the fridge, around your bed, don't forget one in the car and have some as a screensaver on your phone. You can make a few and get your phone to switch them around for you. Maybe you want to record yourself saying them and listen to them during a morning or evening walk or on your way to work.

Focus on positive thoughts with journaling

I suggest a notebook for daily journaling. It can be as basic or pretty as you like. In the mornings take a couple of minutes to write. You can write in bullet points if you like. The practice is to lift your mindset and to start chipping away at your fears. Do it on a daily basis so that you get used to thinking in this way.

My clients use my simple journaling for birth method:

- Take the most negative thought you've had today and turn into into its direct opposite - these will become add to your positive affirmations - collect them and swap them around as you go along

- Write a list of gratitude- I just write ten things I am grateful for every day and as I write them I feel the gratitude, I encourage you to do the same, it is amazing for a positive mindset, but also writing from that place of gratitude and feeling it, helps you in manifesting your intentions for your birth. It embeds your goal and so all the actions you take every day and in your interactions with others will lead you there

- Write out your perfect birth as if it is happening right now or has just happened - you can write bullet points - focus on how you feel

If you have other children or if you are currently feeling a lot of pressure at work, I know this can feel like something else to do. That's not the point, this is not meant to be an added chore but rather a positive action you look forward to every day. It doesn't have to take long at all either. You are not entering a handwriting competition or a spelling contest, just go for it. If mornings are tough, do it before bed. Why not get a Rite In The Rain waterproof pad and write in the bathtub for instance (I haven't tried the shower myself yet, by hey...). Be creative and have fun with it.

Meditation

Like deep breathing, meditation is also part of a traditional Hatha Yoga session. It is usually enjoyed after movement practice and it is called Yoga Nidra.

Yoga nidra simply means yogic sleep. It's a state of staying awake whilst sleeping. Sounds confusing? Well, it simply describes you practising to still your body and your mind whilst remaining conscious. The focus here is on the word 'practice'. To fully be able to dwell in that space of consciousness where you have no distracting messages from your body or your mind is a journey. You get the occasional glimpse of it and then you learn to extend the time you spend there. As soon as you think 'Yessss!!! I got it' you are out of it. So look at your meditation practice as a fun game you have. Don't be hard on yourself if you find this a chore at first, boring even. That's fine. I promise you that after a few attempts you'll start to truly embrace this time of stillness.

This is a practice of self enquiry and you learn a lot about your tendencies. Where do your thoughts tend to drift? Where is it that your body draws your attention to? Where is the tension, where do you experience aches and pains. What part of your body wants to fidget? Just notice it.

Over time you will develop the skill to observe your thoughts and the messages from your body without attachment, eventually stilling your body entirely and therefore giving your thinking mind a break. You can use your meditation practice to positively reinforce an intention.

Your meditation can incorporate your deep breathing practice for labour and for breathing your baby down and you can remind yourself of your affirmations whilst you are deeply relaxed.

Try to make time for this a few times a week or even daily before going to sleep and you will soon observe the benefits of it. Your baby, too, will benefit from your sense of calm and connection. I recommend that you follow a guided relaxation to prepare for your labour. Check out the guided relaxation draft in the next chapter. This is for your birth partner to read out to you or alternatively you can record it for yourself and listen to it on your headphones. Using the same relaxation in labour can be an 'anchor'. Anchors are reminders of situations we were deeply relaxed in. They can be smells, sounds, the voice of a loved one or specific words. Your body remembers being deeply relaxed when those words were spoken to you and therefore you'll relax more quickly in labour hearing those words.

Check out my favourite sound bath on YouTube to provide a relaxing background sound for your meditation, I have linked it in the bonus materials.

Typically, in a meditation practice, you would lie down on your back. However, lying on your back in late pregnancy can make you feel dizzy and faint. In that case you can lie on your side on a yoga mat or in your bed, with a leg draped over a bolster (couch cushions work well for this) or with a good supportive pillow between your knee and lower leg and one to drape your arm over (again, raid the couch cushions – the big ones that you sit on or lean against) You can also set yourself up in a semi reclined pose with your feet flat on the floor or your legs out straight hip width apart like my beautiful client Susan did in the photo below. Be sure to wear loose, comfortable clothing and to bring a blanket because your temperature will drop in relaxation. Which side you lie on for this 10-15 minute practice doesn't really matter. Go with what feels good for you and your baby. Many women tell me 'oh the baby hates it when I lie on my right side/left side'. Find what feels good for both of you.

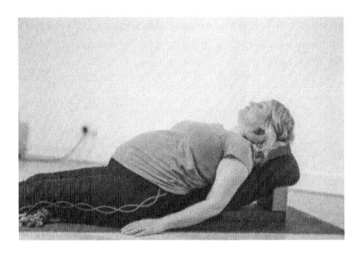

Now having considered how to prepare for your meditation practice, go to your space, turn off your phone and get comfortable. Make sure you won't be disturbed for a while and either get your earplugs in or get your partner to guide you in relaxation. This can feel awkward at first but with a bit of getting used to, this can be a loving and relaxing time for you both. Knowing your partner's voice as an anchor for calm will be great for keeping you calm in labour. You might even use the same script that you have practised through pregnancy. Learning how to help you relax is a great way for your partner to be involved and hands on during labour. Remember this is just a suggested script, again, make it relevant to you, use your own affirmations or write an entirely different script. Don't be afraid to be creative.

Relaxation script with deep breathing practice

This is for your birth partner to read to you:

(Birth partner, read this out slowly and in a calming voice. Make sure you give your partner plenty of time to observe the breath for instance. Watch her and pace yourself as you move through this script. It helps if you breathe with her. It'll give you an idea of how long to pause in between prompts. Don't read out anything in brackets, these are cues and instructions for you. You can play the Sound Bath or your favourite sounds on a low volume in the background as you speak. Tunes without lyrics work best for this)

Script:

'You are getting ready for your relaxation now, make any last adjustments that you need to make in order to feel comfortable. Lengthen your spine and your neck, drop your shoulders back and down and rest back in your comfortable position. (pause for a moment and watch)

If it feels right to do so, let your eyes close.

Now draw your attention to your breath, the inhale - the turn of the breath - the exhale - the return of the breath - four parts to each breath cycle. (wait and watch for at least one cycle of breath, watch your own breath for a cycle or two then move on and continue to read the script)

Each time you are breathing in think - I am breathing in -

Each time you are breathing out, think - I am breathing out - '

(Pause and allow your partner three to five cycles of breath, observing and enjoying the relaxation yourself)

'Now with your next breath cycle, I would like you to introduce a count of three as you breathe in and a count of six as you breathe out'

(this can be adapted to your partner's level of comfort with the yogic breath, just lengthen or shorten it accordingly. Wait for three to five breath cycles, it can be really helpful for your partner if you count her in for the first cycle of breath and then leave her to count at her own pace. After three to five cycles of breath move on to read the script)

'Keep paying attention to your natural breathing for a moment, letting go of the count. Just stay with your breath, watch it ebb and flow.

As you are breathing, try to let go of any thoughts that enter your mind. Just acknowledge them and then let them go. No need to stay attached to any thought, just let them float off, stilling your thinking mind more and more. And as you are paying attention to your breath, notice that you become more and more relaxed'

(Pause and watch for two to three breath cycles)

And now that you are in this relaxed space you are open to really hearing these affirmations:

I am strong

I am relaxed knowing that my body opens perfectly when it's time for my baby to emerge

My body is soft

My baby is wise and knows how to be born

I am at peace trusting my baby

I am confident trusting my body and its ancient wisdom

I am capable

I love my baby

I am grateful that for my baby and for the power to bring new life to this earth

My baby is safe

I am safe

Labour is like my breath - sensations ebb and flow

My baby is carried to me by my breath, I can breathe my baby

out' (add as per your preference)

(Pause and perhaps turn up the tune you have picked - allow for a few minutes of stillness, watch your partner and tune into the relaxation yourself, take the opportunity to feel connected to your baby - after five to ten minutes read on in the script, gently taking your partner out of the relaxation).

In a few moments your relaxation will be complete.

Bring your awareness back to the here and now.

Notice yourself in this room, on this bed. Become aware of where your body touches the sheet.

Now bring some movement into your body.

Wriggle your fingers, your toes.

Once you are ready to do so, open your eyes.

Gently bring yourself into a seated position.

Bring your hands together in front of your heart space.

Take the deepest breath you have taken all day.

Breathe out.

Namaste.'

Namaste is how a yoga nidra meditation is usually concluded. We hold our hands in prayer and say the word 'Namaste'. Namaste simply means 'I bow'. Sometimes it is translated as 'I bow to you' or as 'The Divine in Me Bows To The Divine in you'. It is a greeting that acknowledges our connection to the divine source and to each other and I particularly love it when guiding pregnant families in relaxation. It's a gesture that encircles all of creation and therefore I think it is a perfect way of acknowledging the little one in the womb. If you are not comfortable with it you can conclude your relaxation in whichever way feels right to you. A simple thank you or whatever you like to say to each other can conclude your relaxation practice just the same and if you want to say nothing, just do that. This is your time, you do you!

Build your village - ask for the help you need

Ever heard the expression 'it takes a village'?

Well, truthfully, it does! Bringing a child into the world is a big life transition and as such, traditionally, this would have been witnessed and supported by the female members of the community. But today pregnancies have become a lonely business. Our friends and family members are tied up in busy jobs. Our female elders often don't have great experiences to share about birth. Postpartum often leaves mothers to fend for themselves once the big rush of visitors has ceased, you are expected to be on your feet within days, hours even. Birth and postpartum have lost their traditions of allowing the new family to huddle for a few weeks to integrate the new human.

In this landscape, you may be lacking the caring support from the outside that we need to prepare for this transition to motherhood.

Pregnancy is an invitation to look at your innermost self, explore your own journey, engage with how you were born, connect with your journey on a deeper level. How does it all lead to where you are now? Take the opportunity to explore the thoughts you choose and engage with them. Make time for journaling, do your letting go technique, meditate, breathe and…if you feel really stuck, ask for help!

Talking about giving birth with a pregnancy and birth coach in a group of other like minded mamas gives you a sense of community and you get to ask questions (contact me to find out about my online program or if you are local to Northern Ireland come to my R.O.A.D. To Birth classes). It can also be really helpful to talk about what's on your mind with a family member or friend.

You may want a more tailored approach to your specific circumstance to help you on your fact finding mission. You can enquire about any of my services by via https://www.essentiallybirth.com/contact-sevensecrets

For lingering fears, EFT (emotional freedom technique) or 'tapping' sessions can be helpful, you can find a practitioner near you by following the link in the bonus materials (https://www.essentiallybirth.com/sevensecretsbonuspage).

To work with more deeply rooted fears, you can use EMDR therapy (rapid eye movement therapy), again you can find a link to an international list of practitioners in the bonus materials. If you are struggling with a previous birth experience, three step rewind sessions can be helpful, again, there's a link in the bonus materials to help you find a practitioner.

There are very rare occasions when women find that they need to turn to care providers for medical support with a true phobia of birth and very very rarely pregnancy and postpartum can trigger a psychotic episode. If you feel that you are not coping at all with low mood, fear, anxiety or depression, please speak to your care provider. This is outside of the remit of R.O.A.D. To Birth.

O - Overcome Obstacles

What Obstacles?

Your obstacles to deciding to go after the birth you want for you and your baby can be internal and external and you can work at overcoming both.

Internal obstacles have to do with your mindset, your attitude and willingness to communicate your choices with care providers and family. They can also have to do with your overall health. Overall health can be controlled to an extent with nutrition and lifestyle changes, however some health issues may be ones that you deal with in the A - Acceptance step of the R.O.A.D. to birth system and we will talk about that more

Have you already encountered any situations that you perceive as obstacles to your dream birth scenario?

If so, write them down.

In the next few sections of the book we will explore possible obstacles where you may not suspect them. I recommend that you take notes as you read and then go to the sections in the evidence and decision making section that apply to you.

Internal obstacles

Procrastination

We have all been there. You know that something needs done and you'll do it ...tomorrow. Tidy, get fit, eat better, drink more water, look up those birth stats for your local hospitals and midwife services, do your deep breathing practice...can you think of what yours are?

I can be a master at procrastination when it comes to housework. You should see the state of my home sometimes, I even occasionally manage to give our living room area a teenage bedroom vibe, honestly! The thing that always gets me, though, is how easy it is to *just* tidy, it takes about 15 minutes of my time. Just put things where they go, it really is as simple as that, and it's absolute magic, too. I feel great after it. So I have now adapted a little mantra in my head.

'Don't put it down, put it away!' It's been simple but it makes a huge difference to how I manage my tendency to procrastinate tidying.

Generally I find nutrition, breathwork and movement relatively easy at this stage but it wasn't always like this, in fact getting me to move my body for exercise was a tall order. Most of my old friends are utterly surprised at my five year love affair with weight training and yoga. So what changed? I prioritised movement and health and made a little time for it every day. Initially it was a chore, definitely but I decided to obey the thought 'it's time for a walk, yoga, the gym' every time. And then it became a habit. So, if you are currently feeling that there are things you need to tackle, decide to obey the specific thought right there and then and do it. If you really can't do it right now, write it down and do it immediately when you are free.

Make a list of all the things you 'need to do' to get ready for giving birth. Write them down, decide to do them and then do them. If you feel overwhelmed, put them in an order of priority. I like to use the Eisenhower method of time management. You think of things that are important and urgent. This type of thing in the context of your pregnancy would be when you notice a symptom that really worries you. It's important that you act and you need to act immediately - it's an important thing that's also urgent like putting out a fire. Next you think of things that are important but are not urgent. These are the things that we like to put off. Things that can move us along in our personal development for instance. These things tend to have a deadline but we put them off. Studying for an exam or writing an essay are good examples. In the context of your pregnancy, these are your birth prep activities. It's going to yoga, it's doing your deep breathing, it's taking the time to think of your affirmations.

Then think of things that are not important but urgent. These are the random immediate distractions like a phone ringing or a knock at the door. It feels urgent but it's likely not important. Finally there are things that are not important and not urgent. That's netflix, scrolling on instagram, checking your phone for notifications or reading a book. The easiest way of writing these down is to just divide an A4 page into four quadrants and write 'urgent' and 'non-urgent' into the columns at the top and 'important' and 'not important' into the rows at the side. Then organise your to do list accordingly and assess where you tend to spend your time. Generally we tend to spend a lot of time in the not important or urgent quadrant and that's where you can find the time for the important but not urgent quadrant.

Your physical health

Our physical health is part luck and part behaviour. In the context of exploring our internal obstacles I will speak to the part that is based on health behaviours. The luck part will be revisited in the A- Accept what you can't control chapter.

I would suggest that many harmful health behaviours are based on addictions.

I am immediately thinking of smoking here. Smoking is associated with many adverse health outcomes for you and your baby. If you are currently smoking, ask your provider if you can be referred to get some help with stopping. This will be the biggest positive change you can make in your pregnancy and you will have a great sense of achievement which usually benefits your mood too.

There are other comforts that we may be addicted to. Working on those can have an immediate positive impact on your and your baby's health.

- Poor diet, sugar and comfort foods

- Screen time (and the associated sitting)

- A generally sedentary lifestyle

- Harmful thought patterns

If you are ticking more than one box here, please be kind to yourself. Tackle one habit at a time and celebrate your achievements, there's nobody perfect out there. Pick the habit that you think you can change or the one you think will have the most impact on your life and deal with it first.

In general, becoming more connected to your body by checking in with yourself frequently via meditation and deep breathing and listening to the messages you get from your body will gradually shift you towards a healthier lifestyle. A regular yoga practice honours your physical, mental and spiritual bodies and can be super helpful in letting go of unhelpful habits. Sign up to one of my zoom yoga sessions using the link https://www.essentiallybirth.com/zoom-yoga-sevensecretsreaders.

Do you suffer from a version of 'nice-girl-syndrome'?

Many people struggle with nice girl programming. The term nice girl syndrome was coined by the American psychotherapist Beverly Engel. Beverly is an advocate for women healing from the effects of abusive relationships. She has written a series of books one of which is called 'The Nice Girl Syndrome: Stop Being Manipulated and Abused -- and Start Standing Up for Yourself'. I am bringing this up here because entering maternity care is entering into a relationship with your care providers. Because of the nature of pregnancy and birth the type of relationship you enter will concern areas of intimacy and therefore there is potential for harm. The more aware you are of your boundaries and how well you can communicate those boundaries, the more consciously you can enter into your relationship with your care providers.

What I am alluding to here, is this:

You do the exercises in this book, you identify what you want for yourself and your baby, you've even accepted those things that you can't control and you are at an appointment with your midwife or obstetrician.

You have looked at the wider evidence and you know you don't want a certain intervention or that you would like a certain intervention (maybe an elective caesarean). You state your preference and now you are confronted with the hospital protocol. Your provider is trying to change your mind. You are in a strange environment, not on your own turf, and you came to this appointment on your own.

Are you likely to stand your ground or are you likely to comply?

Be honest with yourself about your tendencies and also have a plan about how you would get the information you need in order to make a truly informed choice? There's the possibility that maybe your provider is offering you the *right* option after all, of course. Will you ask questions, will you listen to your instinct, will you ask for more time? Will you get angry? What will you do?

Observe your tendencies with love and compassion. It's not easy to ask for something that others don't agree with, especially if you are on your own. Adrenaline can get in the way of effective communication, too.

Here's another scenario:

You have chosen to give birth at home and you are telling your mum. She thinks it's irresponsible and she wants you to go to hospital. Or…maybe you want a homebirth and your partner wants you to go to hospital. What are you going to do and how are you going to feel about it? Will you comply and suppress any gut feelings and thoughts that come up telling you that you are making the wrong choice or are you going to stand your ground? How will you communicate? Can you do it from a calm and assertive place, without getting emotional or are you likely to flip your lid. If your opposite flips their lid, how do you deal with that kind of situation? How will you feel knowing that you are doing something a loved one doesn't agree with? Can you still get the support you need?

I told you pregnancy is a great time for getting to know yourself! Take a moment to explore and enquire with yourself, maybe even pause and journal on the question:

Am I A 'Good Girl'?

Challenging your internal obstacles consistently is part of learning to 'Do The Work'.

Your inner obstacles are yours to address. You are in full control of your own behaviours and I am here to invite and motivate you to prepare for your baby's birth by fostering love and connection to yourself so that you can advocate for yourself and your baby in truth.

Are You In?

External obstacles

At this moment in time I am looking at birth with a focus on how you will potentially experience giving birth. We will talk about the practical implications of different choices and their potential advantages and disadvantages later in the book. So when I now present to you that the obstacles to experiencing your dream birth are almost exclusively rooted in medical model of birth I am not suggesting that all interventions are always bad or that everyone should always have a planned caesarean birth without further conversation but I am giving you an idea as to how hospital policy can throw you off course.

If it is a physiological, natural birth you are dreaming of, the obstacles present themselves in the focus on risk in the medical model of birth paradigm. It is so deeply ingrained in our society that it is everywhere. You have now started to work on your internal emotional landscape, so you are taking control of this for yourself, but the people around you may never have explored their fears of pregnancy and birth or started to question what those fears are based on.

External obstacles relate to the fears of other people you are in contact with. Your friends and family may have come to believe that birth needs to be institutionalised for it to be safe. You will encounter their fears as your belly expands and it can be hard work not to make their fears your own.

The more you know, the more you will be able to trust your own intuition and judgement.

You might also encounter midwives and doctors within the medical maternity system who are fully invested in the medicalised birth narrative and who are not providing you with any perspective on the guidelines. This really depends on your area. You could encounter only midwives and doctors who will carefully outline to you all the data they know, help you put it in perspective and make it meaningful for you and then go all out on supporting your choice even if it is out of guideline. I have seen both and I have personally been very lucky to work around people who take the latter approach. However, I also hear from women who are not given objective data and who don't feel supported in making an informed choice.

One of my clients last week met a doctor who told her she was 'very high risk'. The problem was that my client was looking for support for a homebirth and this was out of guideline for her circumstances. She asked what 'very high risk' meant and the answer was: 'You've had a caesarean section before'. My client said that she knew that but really, what was the 'very high risk'. The doctor said that she was 'at 'a high risk of stillbirth'. My client still wasn't happy with the answer and said, 'okay, what is my risk of stillbirth at home compared to coming to hospital. Can you give me statistics on that?' The doctor replied by saying 'I am only going by guideline'. This client had to pull all the stops to get her homebirth.

Meantime another client was supported in her choice for a homebirth after a previous caesarean section by the most amazing team who made every effort to support all of her choices. This team did all the behind the scenes work for out of guideline care without my client even knowing that there is an administrative element to this and without ever feeling any sense of judgement from her care providers.

She ultimately got the same information as my first client. She was asked to consider the additional risk that her caesarean section posed but it was packaged in a much more balanced and compassionate way. Her doctor told her that her specific risk factor was that she had a 1/200 chance of a uterine rupture. She had it explained to her that if this happened at home, then she and her baby would need help urgently and that there was no guarantee that she would arrive in hospital on time to avoid the worst possible outcome. She engaged with this statistic and she asked if there would be any warning signs. She was told, yes, you would likely feel pain across the scar but, again, there was no guarantee. My client felt that on balance the added feeling of safety in her own home and the increased chance of having a natural birth and the long term benefits of this for any possible future children outweighed the 1/200 risk of a uterine rupture. She also decided she would transfer promptly if she had any scar pain at all or if her midwives had the slightest concern about the baby's well being in labour.

Both of these women went on to have a homebirth with no problem, however the first woman felt that she had to fight the whole way through her pregnancy. This happened in different geographical areas, so you can see that it is worth doing some leg work before you decide where you'll have your baby.

I also have an example of a client who wanted a planned caesarean birth that was not medically indicated. She had had two babies before and both of those babies were born without complication and yet, this time she just had a gut feeling that she wanted a caesarean section. She wasn't afraid of birth itself and she knew how a caesarean birth was putting her and her baby at a statistical disadvantage when compared to a vaginal birth and yet she just had a gut feeling that that's what was best. She couldn't rationalise it and couldn't really explain it either. She had a doctor who, again, made sure that she understood fully all the implications of her choice and then facilitated it.

I will say that in general it tends to be easier to convince practitioners in the medical model of care to do something out of guideline than not to do something out of guideline. In my observation and experience negotiating a hands on approach is easier than negotiating a hands off approach. This is due to the underlying belief within maternity systems that birth is only normal in hindsight and that there are many dangers in the process if it is left 'unmanaged'. For instance, induction of labour rates have soared in the last decade despite the fact that there is no conclusive evidence to suggest that this actually keeps babies any safer. There are now more 'risk factors' than a decade ago which has contributed to more and more interventions. This is why this chapter focuses mostly on how the medical industrial model of birth can throw you off the path for a natural birth very quickly if you don't prepare and anticipate certain conversations.

You'll be able to read more about the routine screening tests and interventions in pregnancy, labour and birth in the chapters relating to each intervention in the evidence and decision making section. You'll be able to read in detail what the rationale is for offering them to you and what the potential benefits are in accepting them. You'll also read about how they can throw you off the path to a physiological birth and what the potential disadvantages could be in accepting them.

In order to give you a balanced picture on each of the interventions, I am leaning on data from various sources. I suggest that you read those chapters that apply to you in pregnancy and all the chapters for labour and birth so you can write your birth plan.

Look at this section in the book to identify possible obstacles and also to recognise those things that you will have to accept, things that are not in your power to change.

Routine care offered in pregnancy

More than likely, by the time you have picked up this book, you are already engaged in maternity care in some shape or form.

If you are based in the UK and you have completed your 12th week of pregnancy, I imagine that you have had a booking appointment with your midwife. A booking appointment is what you call the first appointment in your pregnancy. Typically this happens in antenatal clinics in the community or in a maternity hospital. You can refer yourself to your midwife, you don't need your family doctor to do it.

If you are not based in the UK, you will still find this section of the book useful because I am drawing from evidence from around the world when exploring the various topics. Check out the evidence and decision making section for a discussion of the evidence for the aspects of care outlined below.

The main purpose of your initial appointment from the point of view of your midwife or doctor is to do the risk assessment outlined below.

At your initial assessment or 'booking appointment' you'll be assessed as follows:

· Whether you are at an increased risk of developing a blood clot - you'll be offered injections of enoxaparin

· Whether you are at an increased risk of developing high blood pressure or preeclampsia - you'll be offered low dose aspirin

· Whether you are at an increased risk of developing diabetes in pregnancy - you'll be offered a glucose tolerance test (GTT)

· Whether you are at an increased risk of developing anaemia in pregnancy - you'll be offered iron tablets in pregnancy

· Whether your baby is at risk of being growth restricted - you'll be offered serial ultrasound scans

· You can have your bloods checked for HIV, Rubella, Syphilis and Hepatitis B

· You can have your blood group checked and you can be monitored for atypical antibodies in your blood

· Your urine can be sent for screening for Group B strep and other infections

· You can have a 'booking scan' and a due date can be calculated

Tests and prophylactic pharmaceutical medicines are offered in accordance with this assessment.

After this initial assessment you will get a care plan. You can have midwife led care, meaning that you see midwives at every appointment or you can have a care plan that involves seeing midwives and the obstetric doctor at certain stages. Depending on risk factors, you can also have a care plan where you see the obstetricians at each appointment.

If you have been offered a glucose tolerance test, aspirin or enoxaparin injections at your first appointment, you can read about the evidence for each of these screening tests under the respective headings in the evidence and decision making section . You'll also find information on the rationale for the blood tests and urine testing.

Routine care offered throughout pregnancy regardless of your care plan:

- You can have your urine monitored for urinary tract infections and signs of preeclampsia

- You can have your blood pressure checked at each visit

- You can have your belly measured with a tape measure from around 26 weeks or you can have serial scans

- You can decide whether you want to give birth in the hospital, in a midwife led unit or at home attended by a midwife

- You'll be offered membrane sweeps and induction of labour in line with your risk assessment and the associated guidelines

Find the evidence to help you with making informed choices about your care in the evidence and decision making section. For instance, if you have been offered Enoxaparin injections in pregnancy, go to the section 'Are you at risk of developing a blood clot' to help you decide if you want to go ahead with them and so on.

Let's take a look at labour and birth next.

Routine interventions in labour and during birth

You'll maybe wonder why I describe all aspects of routine care in labour and around the time of birth as interventions. The reason is that I am comparing our routine care system directly to a 'desert island birth'.

I am not placing any value on either way of giving birth. The important thing for you to know is that you are free to choose whether you want each and every single aspect of care offered to you. There's no right or wrong way of doing this. It's important that you get to know yourself well enough to know what makes you feel safe and then communicate it to your care providers. In the evidence and decision making section you will find each aspect of care explained and you will see the protocols and evidence that inform midwifery practice in the NHS so that you can make an informed choice about all parts of your care.

- Leaving your home to go to a hospital or birth centre

- Paracetamol or co-codamol

- Foetal heart monitoring, possibly with a cardio tocograph (CTG)

- Routine observations (blood pressure, temperature, your heart rate)

- Partograph - sets a time frame

- Vaginal examinations

- Bladder Care

- Pain relief

Possible interventions in labour and birth

- Starting a partograph and observing the 'three stages of labour'

- Prescribed positions rather than moving instinctively

- 'Active pushing'

- Hands on the perineum (MPOP - manual protection of the perineum)

- Episiotomy (a cut of your perineal muscles)

- Instrumental birth

- Caesarean birth

Interventions once your baby is born

You:

- Active management of third stage (birth of the baby's placenta)

- Suturing

The baby:

- Weighing

- Hat

- Armbands

- Vitamin K

- Managed feeding

·   Possibly a transfer to a postnatal ward and your partner is asked to leave

Here it is not always *just* the midwives who can disrupt the process. What is your priority after the birth? How soon do you feel you would want to spread the news? I often see birth partners on the phone to their relatives as soon as the baby is born, placenta still attached. I have also seen mothers on the phone at this stage and whilst I totally get this, especially in times of restrictions to bringing your mum as another birth partner for instance, it is also you relating out rather than soaking up these moments as a new family and allowing your body the time to complete the birth. Take a moment to talk about this with your birth partner. The birth is not complete until the placenta is born and physiologically your ancient blueprint still likes peace and quiet at this time to finally release the biggest wave of oxytocin you can ever experience in life and therefore complete the process of birth safely and without complication.

Pregnancy-Labour-Birth-Postpartum are a continuum. If a natural birth free from any intervention is important to you, go back to the chapter 'Understanding Physiological/Natural Birth' and read through that again to remind yourself of the physical and hormonal processes in pregnancy and birth. They'll be initiated by your body and they are available to you at any point in your pregnancy and birth. I have listed the routine interventions here because they can potentially present themselves as obstacles to a natural birth if you fall out of the expected norm. As I have stated earlier, it appears to me that it is generally easier to ask for an intervention like a caesarean birth out of guideline or to make a case for an induction of labour than it is to decline an intervention.

Refer to the evidence and decision making section in order to read about how the interventions I have listed above are implemented within the medical obstetric care model, the rationale for them and how they could interfere with the natural continuum. You can pick and choose to read only the ones that apply to you or you can read them all.

Depending on your circumstances, guidelines associated with each of the observations and screening tests offered to you can put an induction of labour on the cards or take a homebirth or midwife led unit birth off the cards. They can potentially introduce more anxiety and on the other hand you might feel reassured by them. As you will see in the various chapters in the evidence and decision making section , there is no right or wrong answer, your choices about whether to accept or decline each aspect of pregnancy and labour care and your choice of place of birth are deeply personal and you can advocate for yourself if you would like to avail of out of guideline care.

Once you have explored the topics that are relevant to you, come back to the list of routine interventions when writing your birth plan so that you can state your preferences for all of the intervention points.

If you are not sure whether you are deemed 'high' or 'low risk' ask your care provider. I would suggest that you ask for the specific risk factors (if any) to be outlined to you so that you can take a deep dive into the topics starting at the evidence and decision making section and then expanding your reading accordingly.

Now take a moment to make a list of all your potential and actual obstacles so that you can start at making plans to overcome them. Your internal ones can often be tackled in the same way you address any fears you might have identified. The external ones will fall into two categories: you choose to accept them or you work at overcoming them.

Move on to the next chapter when you have made your list.

A - Accept What You Can't Control

Accepting what you can't control takes some work and reflection. The messaging in our society suggests to us that we can control pretty much everything. We are less and less prepared to accept that sometimes things just are what they are.

We can choose to struggle, beat ourselves up, beat others up, complain about 'the system' and 'those midwives and doctors', we can blame people for 'how they made us feel' and we may even have a point but we can't control it. Ultimately we are on our own to decide how we deal with it.

The only factor we can really ever control is our response to each situation presenting itself.

There are things we don't get to decide no matter how much we would like to.

You might have been born with a disability or a heart condition for instance, or a tragedy in your life has permanently changed your body. Your pregnancy journey will differ from routine care. It is important to remember that you know your body best and that you can choose in and out of elements of care like everyone else.

In this chapter we will discuss those pregnancy situations where your options truly are limited. We will talk about how you can work at accepting those things you can't control.

Some rare pregnancy complications that dictate an elective caesarean

In the context of birth, there are a couple of (rare) scenarios that only leave you with a caesarean section as a way forward.

A planned caesarean birth is vital for your and your baby's survival in the case of a major placenta praevia. That's when the placenta is attached over the cervix and labouring in this case would lead to profound bleeding putting your and your baby's lives at risk (if you are reading this with a 'low lying placenta' at your 19 week scan, please know that this resolves in 90% of cases. Major placenta previa only occurs in around 1/200 pregnancies and is more likely if you have had a caesarean before). This is a scenario where a caesarean section really is your only option. You can change course and start making plans around having a positive experience at your baby's emergence by caesarean section. If you are having trouble with accepting this, your affirmation and journaling practice could include something like this: 'I am grateful that I have caesarean sections available to me.' or 'This is how my baby is choosing to be born'.

The other rare scenario is when your baby continues to lie sideways. There are a few things you can try to figure this out with your baby in pregnancy but by the time you go into labour, you really need your baby to go head or bum first in order to be born.

There are a few very rare emergency scenarios that can knock your plans, and your work on accepting those generally starts after the baby is born. This can be a process. Generally, it tends to be easier if you have felt fully informed leading up to the situation and you can integrate your experience. If you have been through something like this and you are struggling, please reach out to your care providers. Generally there are services to help you with this. You can also seek a birth rewind session often provided by doulas. Sign up for the bonus materials for help with finding a practitioner.

If you are reading this never having had a scan, look out for any bleeding in pregnancy and get in touch with your care provider so that you can decide if you want to be checked out for placenta previa.

What can and can't you control otherwise?

When it comes to your decision making about aspects of your care, acceptance can take different forms for different people.

For instance you might go and read the various bits of evidence presented to you in the evidence and decision making section and decide to go with hospital guidance. You have asked for the rationale for offering you interventions when you didn't know and you are happy with the explanations. On balance you would rather trust your midwife or doctor than make decisions out of guideline where you have to trust yourself to make the right choice. You accept whatever interventions are offered to you and accept that in doing so your chances of having an induction of labour or a caesarean birth are whatever the statistics at your local hospital say. You read up on the practical aspects of inductions of labour and caesareans and you work on overcoming any fears specific to those. You come to fully accept that path. On the flip side of that you feel relief that the midwives and doctors carry most of the responsibility and you can relax fully into your experience.

Or, you might read the materials and decide to opt out of aspects of care guidelines. Maybe you decline a specific prophylactic drug in your pregnancy or maybe you opt for an out of guideline homebirth attended by midwives. You accept that you may have to engage in some uncomfortable conversations and that you will be reminded of risk factors along the way. You accept that your care providers will have to continue to offer care according to their guidelines and policies and that you will be engaged in conversations at any point a situation changes and a certain care pathway would now be recommended. You also accept responsibility for your informed decisions and the potential advantages as well as disadvantages of your choices. You accept that you can't control the guidelines themselves and the fact that your care providers are bound to offer care to you in line with them. You anticipate the conversations and you take on board new factors for consideration as situations evolve. For labour, you might hire a doula as an advocate so that you can stay in your zone and let your birth hormones do their thing.

It may also be that you only trust yourself. You see birth as a physiological and sacred process that does not comply with the normal parameters as defined by the guidelines within the medical obstetric system. You accept that you can't control the guidelines or the fact that midwives and doctors are bound by them but you choose that they are not for you. You are not willing to engage with any aspect of this at all and you have decided not to place yourself in proximity of people who will offer care based on the guidelines because you feel that it is too much work to swim against the current within these parameters. You decide to give birth outside the system and you accept that the price of not outsourcing and deferring any aspects of your decision making to midwives or doctors is that all responsibility for yourself and your baby lies with you. You accept the unknowns that come with this choice and also the possible backlash and stigma that comes with stepping away from the cultural norm.

All of those scenarios are 100% valid choices. We are exchanging varying aspects of control over our bodily autonomy against outsourcing some of the sense of responsibility for our own and our baby's wellbeing. So, our perception of 'accepting what we can't control' will be different in each scenario. This is our prerogative and it is a deeply personal choice. On balance the perceived advantages of each course has to outweigh the perceived disadvantages and our choices have to fit into our values and beliefs. One way of seeing it is that all of us need to work on finding acceptance for the event that we have to deal with one or more of the disadvantages.

Regardless of the path we choose, we all have to accept that there are situations where we may need to call for help in the form of a medical intervention even if we didn't want to. Regardless of what your chosen place of birth is, it is a good idea for everyone to identify and let go of those fears specific to hospitals and medical interventions and work on accepting that it is within the realm of possibility that unexpected events occur.

On the other hand, working on accepting that parts of your birth plan that involve medical personnel are dependent on the situation in the hospital or in the community on the day is also important. For instance, you may have to wait for an epidural for some time, so have labour strategies up your sleeve for that situation. Or your community midwife service may be very busy and may have to step down the on call arrangements on the day you need them. All of these scenarios are unlikely but they can happen and it's good to have worked on accepting those types of situations and have a plan B.

Trigger Warning

The next chapter talks about accepting the possibility of losing a child. If you would prefer not to engage with this subject, skip through to the 'How to find acceptance' part.

At this stage I would like to acknowledge that you might be reading this having had the experience of losing a child. If you are walking this walk, I extend my deepest sympathy for you. I want to make sure that you know that you are not alone on this journey. If you haven't already connected with SANDS, I encourage you to reach out. SANDS is a UK-based charity who offer support to parents who have lost a baby in pregnancy or in infancy and there are many local groups and online resources. You can find a link to their website in the reference list.

Accepting the most difficult reality of all:

When we conceive the potential for new life, we also conceive the possibility of losing our child.

This is difficult to read as a parent, particularly when you are only starting out on your journey to parenthood. It is the most frightening thought there is and yet there's nobody and nothing that can take that away from us. We can give birth in hospital, at home, in the Pacific Ocean, in a state of the art obstetric theatre, the potential is always there. We get to choose to either accept this or make all of our decisions based on the fear of it actually happening.

In the German language we describe pregnancy as 'in guter Hoffnung sein' which literally translates as 'being in good hope'. It means you expect everything to go well but you don't take it for granted. I find this a beautiful way of engaging with the full spectrum of what it means to be a parent.

The possibility of losing our child will stay with us for our lifetimes as mothers and as parents. I still have to work with my fears around this too even though my daughter is an adult. And yet, it seems that there is never a time when we are made as acutely aware of it as in pregnancy and birth. The messaging in the media, society as a whole and from medical obstetric care professionals implies that we can prevent this from happening if we just try hard enough. Combined with the concept of informed choice this message places mothers in the hot seat. Pregnant women can feel under pressure from all angles. On one hand we have this ideal image of what birth should be and all the reasons why this is good for ourselves as mothers and on the other hand you have a system whose guidelines suggest that birth is only safe when medically managed… but you chose! The implication that mothers are ultimately responsible for their baby's primal health and their survival by every single choice they make is everywhere. It's a burden a lot of mothers carry and this is a good place for me to let you know that no matter what you do in pregnancy, how well you connect with your baby or how many scans and investigations you go to or don't go to, ultimately and finally whether a baby lives or dies is not for us to control. We can consistently work on safety and birth may become even safer statistically speaking, but some of us will have to walk that painful walk of suffering the loss of a child.

What if we accepted that the possibility of losing our child is there regardless of our choices, nobody can make it go away entirely. That loving our babies and making each decision from a place of true authenticity and love is the best we can do for them. That beyond that we have to hand it over to…god, the universe, chance? Whatever philosophy fits into your values and beliefs is where you can find acceptance.

How freeing would that be? What if we accepted that ultimately we do not get to decide if our child lives or dies. What if we embraced the mantra 'Be Here Now' and stopped worrying about the what ifs. How different would our experience of pregnancy be from this place of acceptance?

Losing your child during pregnancy, birth or in the early postpartum days is the most unlikely thing to happen. It's possible regardless of who you enlist for care and support, and yet, hardly anybody ever encourages you to work at accepting the possibility of loss. So I will be brave and invite you to find acceptance and make space for this possibility so you can let go of fear and make your choices from a place of complete freedom.

From here the choice of opting into interventions is just as free and plausible and perfect as opting out. You'll be able to make your choices from a truly informed place because you can take a step back and you can evaluate the data available to you and enquire with your intuition to come to the choice that is right for you and your baby.

If you want to read more about the statistical likelihood of losing a baby, check out the chapter in the evidence and decision making section. In it I quote statistics from the latest report published by MBRRACE-UK. MBRRACE stands for Mothers and Babies: Reducing Risk through Audits and Confidential Enquiries across the UK and their most recent report collates statistics gathered between January and December 2019. You might find the data reassuring and helpful at gaining perspective.

How to find acceptance

My strategies are very similar to the ones I use for working on letting go of fear. Try to first identify where your locus of trust lies and then deduct what the factors are that you can't control in that context.

Incorporate those factors in your meditation, deep breathing and journaling practice. At the risk of sounding morbid, I also invite you to explore your beliefs around life and death. Your own mortality is a good place to start. Where do your beliefs come from? Are you religious and have your beliefs been given to you as part of your religious beliefs? Can you be courageous and question if they feel right for you? There is a true sense of liberation in letting go of the fear of death. You'll be able to make your choices from a place of calm and trust and you'll be able to access your intuition more easily.

As you know, I am a yogi and for me, listening to the Be Here Now Network Podcast and to Ram Dass in particular has helped me with accepting those things that are out of my control. I have linked the podcast in the bonus materials for ease of access if you want to dip in and you can easily find it online by typing Ram Dass 'Be Here Now' into your search engine.

D - Do The Work (Daily Habits)

Doing the work means to commit to working on recognising and releasing your fears, overcoming your obstacles and accepting what you can't control as part of your daily life.

It also means getting an idea of what the maternity care provision is in your area.

Here's what to do:

- Do the groundwork

- Evaluate your lifestyle habits

- Make a birth plan

- Implement a daily routine

- Ask your birth partner to join you on the R.O.A.D. To Birth

Doing the groundwork

Find out your care provider's statistics and change providers if another option has statistics that are likely to facilitate your dream birth better. You want a waterbirth? Go where they happen a lot! You want a planned caesarean? Go where they happen a lot. Get the big picture and focus on what's important to you.

Here's what to ask:

What's your induction of labour rate?
What's your spontaneous vaginal birth rate?
What is your epidural rate? (this will help you to discern how many of the spontaneous vaginal births are 'desert island births' if that's important to you)
What's your waterbirth rate?
What's your instrumental birth rate?

What's your caesarean section rate?

What's your episiotomy rate?

What's your 3rd and 4th degree tear rate?

What's your rate of haemorrhage?

Do you have a continuity of carer team (where you know your midwife before birth)

Do you have a midwife led unit?

Do you offer homebirth?

What's your transfer rate from midwife led to obstetric led care?

What is your transfer rate of babies to the neonatal unit?

If you are a first time parent, ask the birth related statistic in relation to first time mums. Usually this information is displayed on maternity dashboards and it might be available online. If not, ask at your next appointment and ask who you can ask for it if your midwife doesn't know.

Lifestyle

As you will see in the evidence and decision making section , the screening tools used in maternity care are assessing you against health factors that are out of your control and lifestyle factors. Generally lifestyle factors play part in your overall health and quality of life and making some changes may give you a similar benefit as prophylactic pharmaceutical treatments. In any case, making positive changes in your lifestyle certainly won't do any harm. Doing the work may mean taking a look at any habits you have that impact your health negatively.

Incorporate some daily movement. Movement and diet interventions alone have helped women with pregnancy induced high blood pressure reduce their blood pressure without medication. Switching to a high fibre plant based diet can help you tackle gestational diabetes, so why not choose to incorporate a daily movement practice and choose a diet rich in plants and fibre, avoiding ultra processed foods and sugar. Be proactive to try and keep your risk to a minimum but please speak to your care providers if you are already diagnosed with any pregnancy related or pre-existing condition. Tell them the changes you are intending to make and ask for their input, support and supervision.

What's your diet like?

Do you eat plenty of fruit and veg?
Do you limit your sugar intake?
Do you fall back on prepacked highly processed foods often?
Do you drink fizzy drinks?
What's your tea and coffee intake like?

I suggest having an honest look at your baseline diet right now. If you are up for keeping a food diary for a day to gather some data on your habits, go ahead. You may already have an idea and know where there is room for improvement. I encourage you to do this with love and without judgement. This is not another stick to beat yourself with.

Some tips to make it easy:

- Batch-freeze bags of chopped veg with all the ingredients for a stew or soup and pop it all into a pot or (better still) your slow cooker in the morning. Come home to a nutritious stew.

- Standardise your breakfast, just have two or three fibre rich staple breakfasts. I like overnight oats with lots of chia and sunflower seeds and fruit.

- Have the same dinner on alternate nights. Saves time cooking.

A little goes a long way. If you are currently not happy with your diet, just make a small change and feel the impact. Go gradually and before you know it, you are cooking up a storm of healthy foods. In the long run, your entire family will benefit.

Questions to answer for your birth plan (refer to the evidence and decision making section to decide your preference):

Where do you want to give birth?

Who will be with you?

Would you like a waterbirth?

What method of pain relief would you like to use?

Point out how important it is to you to be mobile and walk around, change position?

Would you like to have routine vaginal examinations as per the hospital protocol?

Would you like to have routine observations in labour and would you like to be monitored with a partograph?

Would you want your waters released by artificial rupture of membranes?

Would you like to be told to 'push'?

Point out whether you would like your midwife to touch your perineum as the baby comes out and would you consent to an episiotomy?

Who discovers your baby's sex (you yourself, your partner or do you want the midwife to call it out)?

When (if at all) does your baby's cord get cut and who cuts it?

What about the birth of your placenta? Do you want an injection or not?

Would you like your baby to be left skin to skin with you at birth?

Do you want your baby weighed and when?

Do you want a hat on your newborn baby?

Do you want your baby to have vitamin K?

Do you want the baby to do a breast crawl or would you like support with breastfeeding?

If you are feeding your baby with formula milk, which milk will it be and who feeds your baby for the first time?

Consider also that you'll likely be offered membrane sweeps and possibly an induction of labour. Know how you feel about those before you go to your appointments from 34 weeks onwards. I highly recommend reading

Dr Sara Wickham's book 'In your own time' to help you with making decisions around induction of labour in different circumstances.

Daily routine

The easiest way to incorporate a five to ten minute breathing practice, a little movement and a meditation practice is to roll out your yoga mat and commit to a short and sweet yoga practice first thing in the morning or before bed. Join me for a 15 minute practice and use it as often as possible. You can find links at the start and the end of the book. Aim to add a longer meditation session two to three times per week over your earphones, if you fall asleep, no worries. Sign up for my bonus materials to access a guided relaxation.

Make it a habit to stretch, maybe in the shower or as you brush your teeth. Make moving through your day fun and find ways to incorporate some simple side body stretches whilst waiting for your kettle to boil, stirring your stew or reaching for your crockery. Be mindful and enjoy it.

Do your deep breathing every time you wait for a bus, sit on the loo, or chill out in front of the tele.

Aim to fit in an after dinner walk when you can. Walking in big strides releases your psoas muscle. The psoas muscle is the muscle that connects your torso to your legs on each side of the body. Your baby moves past in order to engage into the pelvis, so moving it and keeping it nice and subtle in pregnancy and in early labour can help your baby find the way into the pelvis. Walking keeps you active, improves your digestion, gets you into the fresh air, helps you clear your head and adds to a positive mindset.

So, you see, it doesn't have to be another thing to do but rather something that becomes part of your life.

Here's how to structure a 15 - 30 minute daily routine

5 - 10 minute journaling practice

15 - 20 minute yoga practice

Or

5 - 10 minute journaling practice
5 - 10 minute dedicated breathing practice
5 - 10 minute deep relaxation/meditation practice

Check out any thoughts of 'I won't have time' or 'I am too busy' and ask yourself if they are true and what your priority is. What is it you'll be doing instead? Can you steal some time from somewhere? Why are you rushing? How much time do you spend on social media? How much time do you spend with non-nurturing activities? Be kind to yourself and also challenge yourself. Hold yourself accountable.

Would you show up on your wedding day in your jeans and T-shirt because you didn't have time to look for a dress?

Would you order a takeaway because you didn't feel like planning a nice meal for your guests?

Make a decision to prepare for giving birth and then stick to it.

R.O.A.D. To Birth For The Birth Partner

Hello birth partner. If you are going to be present at the birth of this baby, it will be very beneficial for you to do some ground work, too. Whether this is your child, grandchild, niece or nephew or your best friend's baby. The important thing when you step into the birth space is that you yourself are free from fear or at least that you can keep your own emotions regulated so that they don't spill over to your partner or loved one.

What are your fears?

Go to the R - Recognise and release your fears chapter and make it your own. Be honest about what your beliefs are. Sit together and compare notes. Be honest with each other and try not to judge each other for your opinions. Instead be curious and see where you can help each other with data and using the tools in the chapter.

What are your obstacles?

Look for obstacles to supporting your loved one. These can again be internal and external. Are there parts of your birth plan together that involve you? How calm can you stay and how do you have 'good child syndrome'? Are you prepared to advocate for your partner or loved one and can you do it calmly, without aggression? How will you get the information you need in order to help your partner or loved one in their decision making in labour? Are you aware of the birth plan and can you point it out? Do you need to hire a doula to support you both as a couple?

What are the things you need to accept?

Are there any aspects of your partner or loved one's choices that you disagree with and can you accept them?

What work do you need to do?

Is there anything practical you can help with? Can you help with getting some dashboard information from the local maternity care providers? Can you take on some of the cooking? Can you help motivate your partner or loved one to go for a walk or do some yoga with them? Do you smoke and can you stop? Will you read out the relaxation scripts to your partner?

Evidence And Decision Making Section

About this section

In this section I will present the data around individual parts that make up routine maternity care in the UK. It's also the things women most commonly ask me questions about. There's a lot of data and quoting guidelines in here and because of that, there's also a lot of referencing in brackets. You might feel that some of this reads like a university essay or a journal article. I have tried to keep it as engaging as I can whilst endeavouring to give you as big a picture as possible without turning this section into another book.

As more studies get done, evidence changes and therefore recommendations and policy may change. As I said earlier in this book, policy also varies from area to area and I encourage you to ask questions about what common practices and policies are in your area of care. I also want to remind you that no part of this book replaces individual professional midwifery or medical care and advice. It is designed to offer general information only.

TRIGGER WARNING

Because outcomes are largely measured against worst case scenarios, when discussing evidence around interventions the subject of baby loss and illness will weave through parts of this section. Particularly the next section 'about risk and risk factors' speaks about the overall likelihood of you or your baby dying in birth. Again, please know that I truly honour that all of the points of discussion in the next section are not *just* data and that they reflect the lived experiences of women, partners and their wider families. I also know that the health problems we will discuss here are not just terms - like perineal trauma for instance - but they reflect a journey.

This section of the book aims to give you a balanced approach to evidence and guidelines and the wider picture of each consideration. The more evidence there is, the more complex the discussion becomes. You will see that generally (but not always) interventions shift the needle towards better outcomes in relation to the particular risk the intervention aims to reduce. Sometimes those shifts are marginal. You will have to decide if the potential disadvantages are outweighed by the potential advantages.

Because of this complexity and because nobody can predict the outcome, I frequently refer you back to your values, beliefs and inner knowing as well as the data. When I refer you back to yourself, I don't mean to imply that you can predict and prevent worst case scenarios if you just try hard enough. I don't think this is possible. What I do think though is that you know best what's good for you and your baby in a wider sense and I encourage you to trust yourself in making those decisions with confidence.

Some people opt out of all interventions, some people opt into all interventions and others are somewhere in between. In my experience those people who make their decisions consciously and from a place of knowledge tend to be happier with their birth experiences.

I have tried my best to deal with each subject in as sensitive a manner as possible whilst also staying factual. I truly want for you to be able to make fully informed decisions about each aspect of your care. I appreciate how complex this can get and I am here to help you. If you have questions and would like to book an online one-to-one session, you can book an appointment via https://www.essentiallybirth.com/zoom-one-to-one-sevensecrets.

About risk and risk factors

Risk is how the medical profession talks about the possibility of someone getting seriously or dying when a certain condition is identified. Because midwifery has become so deeply embedded into the medical system, midwives use the same language to refer to the *condition* of pregnancy.

Mainstream maternity care will triage you into one of two categories of women:

'High risk' or 'low risk' or, ideally, 'Universal care' and 'additional care' groups of women

Even though the Nursing and Midwifery Council (NMC) Standards (2019) moved away from the terms 'low risk' and 'high risk' in favour of 'universal care' and 'additional care', the term 'risk' still commonly appears in the language directed at pregnant women in most areas. I will continue to speak about understanding risk in various contexts because in my experience in speaking with women in a pregnancy and birth coaching capacity this is the language you are most likely to encounter.

Once a doctor at a maternity conference pointed out that this language presents us with certain limitations because we give a woman with a double lung and heart transplant the same label as we give to a woman who gave birth by caesarean section last year or simply 'goes overdue'. I would credit the doctor but I can't remember his name. He made a good point though.

Until I ended up working as a midwifery sister in the management team of a free standing midwife led unit I was somewhat oblivious to the fact that 'risk assessment' is considered to be one of the most important aspects of a midwife's role.

In hindsight it is glaringly obvious that my employers have always seen my role in that way, but I have never looked at birth as inherently dangerous and so I have always seen the role of a midwife as a guardian of birth physiology rather than a risk assessor.

Your midwife is trained to assess your medical history for factors that are known to increase your or your baby's risk of getting seriously ill or dying when compared to the baseline risk that comes with simply being pregnant or waiting to be born.

According to data gathered between January and December 2019, the overall baseline risk of dying was 4.96/1000 pregnancies for a baby from 22 weeks of pregnancy, at or around the time of birth and up to four weeks of age (MBRRACE, 2021). Data gathered between 2017 and 2019 suggests that the risk of women dying due to childbirth is 8.8/100 000 (MBRRACE, 2021).

I know most mums are not particularly worried for their own life but reading about babies dying is difficult in pregnancy, particularly if you have experienced a loss before. I am truly sorry for this. I want to give you as much information as I can because ultimately this information will show you that pregnancy and birth are inherently safe for both of you. This is important if you ever find yourself making a decision about a suggested intervention, particularly if you wish to advocate for yourself in case you wish to opt out.

I always suggest that you ask for a discussion of your risk in absolute terms rather than in relative terms. Hearing that your risk is 30% increased or double or that the intervention offers 98% protection doesn't give you the information you need to assess it in a meaningful way. Who wouldn't want 98% protection? But what does it actually mean in real data? Lets take your own risk of dying in pregnancy and let's assume there's a circumstance in which it could 'double'. That puts your absolute risk of dying at 17.6/100 000. How worried would you be hearing this data compared to 'your risk of dying doubles if we don't do x,y or z?

I recently coached a couple who had just come out of an antenatal appointment. They walked into the appointment entirely unassuming and walked out with various 'issues' identified at 37 weeks. They were told they were 'putting their baby at risk of stillbirth' by not having an induction of labour at 39 weeks because the woman was over 40. I personally find this implication that the risk only exists if you don't opt for an induction of labour offensive. It undermines women and gaslights them into placing their locus of trust into the hands of the medical apparatus. It is simply not true that induction of labour mitigates all risk to your baby. That doesn't mean that it would be wrong to opt for an induction of labour in this case, it just means that your decision was made without any data but by inducing fear.

When we explored their specific risk for stillbirth together, we found there to be various sources of data. The RCOG (2013) states that at 39–40 weeks of gestation the risk of stillbirth equates to 2 in 1000 for women of 40 years of age or older compared to 1 in 1000 for women younger than 35 years of age. This represents a similar stillbirth risk at 39 weeks of gestation for women over 40 compared to women in their mid 20s at 41 weeks of gestation. This is why, according to the RCOG (2013), induction of labour should be offered around term to women over 40 to prevent late stillbirth. The couple had bought the book 'In your own time' by Dr Sara Wickham. We looked at the chapter on older women and found a detailed discussion on the subject. We learned how difficult it is to determine absolute risk of stillbirth with advanced age because often advanced age can mean that other health factors have developed for the women. Dr Wickham quotes a large study conducted in the Netherlands for the best available data on maternal age and stillbirth. My client found that her absolute overall risk of stillbirth according to this study was 1 in 333 (Wickham, 2021). Now the couple had relevant data at hand to make a choice at the end of their pregnancy, however, they went into labour before they were 'due' and so they never had to.

In every single scenario that arises in your pregnancy, it is entirely justifiable to decide either way. If you have the data you can assess what feels right to you. Ultimately, regardless of how we choose, we do not know what will happen in the future. We don't get to know and we don't get to decide. Allow yourself to be informed by your instincts as well as available data and to make your decision in the context of your own values and beliefs. Please bear with me for a closer look at the data to help you do just that.

In order to put things in perspective for you, I will elaborate on this by referring to the latest data presented by MBRRACE-UK. MBRRACE stands for Mothers and Babies: Reducing Risk through Audits and Confidential Enquiries across the UK. The full report is linked in the reference list in case you would like to read it for yourself.

As I said earlier, your baby's baseline risk of dying in pregnancy or in the early postnatal period (perinatal mortality rate) is 4.96 per 1000 births. This represents babies born from 24 weeks onwards. Overall this rate has dropped from 6.04 in 2013.

The perinatal mortality rate is made up of the stillbirth rate itself (3.35 /1000 in 2019) and babies dying after they were born (1.62/1000 in 2019). Most of all of these babies died before 37 weeks of gestation. The decrease in perinatal mortality is mainly attributed to fewer very premature babies dying after they are born and to a reduction of stillbirth between 37 and 41 weeks (from 1.45 per 1,000 total births in 2015 to 1.17 in 2019). The stillbirth rate at 42 weeks or after was 0.61/1000 babies in 2019.

Mothers dying in pregnancy or birth thankfully is even more unlikely and is 8.8 women per 100 000. I have linked to the summary of the latest MBRRACE - UK report in the bonus materials if you would like to take a look.

Hopefully you find this data reassuring. To me it illustrates how well equipped we are to grow healthy babies and give birth to them.

Any conversations about 'risk' happen in the context of this background data and also in the context of your or your baby's likelihood of suffering serious or life changing injuries. The most commonly measured outcomes for babies are a baby's need for resuscitation, serious infections, sepsis and birth injuries due to lack of oxygen, instrumental births or injuries sustained during a caesarean section. For mums the main reason to become seriously ill are linked to blood loss at birth and infection or sepsis. Life changing injuries can happen in the context of severe injuries to your perineum (the muscular area between your vagina and your anus) or bladder injuries related to the pregnancy itself, the birth or sustained at a caesarean section.

Sadly common public perception of birth is that it is dangerous. This perception often rides on isolated cases. Often such cases involve internal or external investigations, large court settlements and media attention.

This is a really delicate topic because each and every 'outcome' or 'case' represents suffering for a mother and her family and as compassionate humans we want to eradicate this type of heartbreak. The challenge is striking the balance between truly helping and doing harm whilst trying to help.

I have always seen it as my role as a midwife to help women strike that balance because in general clinicians will be keen to stick to hospital policy and they are prone to over-representing the potential benefits of an intervention and underrepresented the potential downsides. I offer zoom consultations for women who are seeking to explore their choices in the context of their own stories. You can book a session via https://www.essentiallybirth.com/zoom-one-to-one-sevensecrets.

In the next sections I will discuss risk in terms of specific routine interventions offered in pregnancy, birth and the immediate postpartum. You can hop and skip chapters that don't apply to you.

Are you at increased risk of developing a blood clot?

Blood clots in your circulation are dangerous and they can cause an embolism. Embolisms can be fatal if they enter the lung, heart or brain tissue. They can block the circulation to these vital organs and can cause a stroke or heart attack or a pulmonary embolism (clot in the lung). Pulmonary embolism (PE) remains one of the leading causes a mum dies in pregnancy or immediately after in the UK today.

Remember that your overall risk of dying in your childbearing year is very low at 8.8/100 000 pregnant women according to the 2019 MBRRACE-UK report. PE was the reason 16% of these women died (MBRRACE, 2019).

Clots can form in pregnancy or afterwards, particularly if you have had a caesarean or an instrumental birth. The practice of offering you Enoxaparin for 7-10 days after a caesarean birth has been common practice in the UK for around two decades. It was first approved for medical use in 1993 (NIH, 2021), however, the practice of offering it during pregnancy was only introduced in 2015 via a guideline issued by the Royal College of Obstetrics and Gynaecologists (RCOG). Enoxaparin is a blood thinning drug and it is used to prevent or disperse blood clots. It is in the group of drugs called low molecular weight heparins.

The risk assessment is complex, assigning points against various risk factors. Factors include whether you have a family history of unprovoked blood clots, whether you are carrying more than one baby, whether you have ever had an unprovoked blood clot yourself, your BMI, how many children you have had, if you smoke, if you have preeclampsia or have had IVF for instance. The factors are scored and you will be offered injections from the first trimester, from 28 weeks, after your baby is born or not at all. The assessment gets repeated mid pregnancy, after you have had your baby or if you are admitted to hospital in pregnancy and Enoxaparin is offered to you accordingly.

How does taking the injections change your risk of developing a blood clot in pregnancy?

Your baseline risk of developing a blood clot in pregnancy is low at 1-2 per 1000 pregnancies (RCOG, 2015).

When it comes to looking at how your risk is reduced, the RCOG looked at people in hospitals and people who have had surgery in the general population where using Enoxaparin was associated with reducing the incidence of a blood clot by 60% for people in hospital for various reasons and 70% after surgery. It was deemed reasonable to assume that a similar reduction in risk would be observed in pregnancy and postpartum (RCOG, 2015).

If you would like to check out the guideline, I have referenced it in the reference list. Also remember to access the bonus materials or quick links to the references I used and all the other extra goodies too.

The guidelines focus on the potential benefit of Enoxaparin.

There is currently no good trial or meta analysis data that compares the overall outcomes for mothers and babies when comparing mothers who use Enoxaparin in pregnancy to mothers who didn't (Jacobson, et al. 2019). All we know is that it is likely to reduce your chances of developing a serious and potentially life threatening complication which occurs 1-2 times per 1000 births by around 60-70%. Therefore the potential benefit of giving Enoxaparin routinely to women with risk factors is considered to outweigh any potential risk to you or your baby.

You will see as we go along that your decisions will ultimately depend on your own assessment of the potential benefit of an intervention versus the potential disadvantages. This is a deeply personal decision, it's nuanced and it depends on your personal values and beliefs and most importantly there's no right or wrong answer.

Are you at an increased risk of developing high blood pressure or pre-eclampsia?

Preeclampsia is a pregnancy condition that affects between up to 8% of pregnancies in the UK (RCOG, 2022). It can be diagnosed in pregnancy, birth or postpartum and although it is mostly mild, it can be life threatening for you and your baby if it is severe.

It is a disorder that increases your blood pressure and in severe cases it can change how your blood is composed and therefore cause other complications. Symptoms are headaches, disturbed vision, pain just below the ribs, vomiting and sudden swelling. Preeclampsia can cause liver problems and kidney problems and it can affect your heart and brain. The exact way it works and exactly how it can be avoided is not known, however, low dose aspirin has been used for the last few years now in order to try and prevent it for women with risk factors.

Aspirin is a non steroidal anti-inflammatory drug (NSAID) and it is most commonly used to reduce temperature and inflammation. It is also used as a prophylactic treatment in various situations in modern medicine, most commonly in the prevention of heart disease (BNF, 2022).

The normal dose of Aspirin (for pain **outside of pregnancy**) is 300-900 mg every 4-6 hours and no more than 4g should be taken in total (BNF, 2022). I just want to make it very clear here, that aspirin is not recommended to treat headaches or other types of pain in pregnancy. In fact the only application in pregnancy is daily low dose aspirin for people who have risk factors for preeclampsia. I am only stating the usual dosage for reference and perspective.

The recommendation to offer low dose Aspirin (75 - 150 mg daily) to women who are more at risk of developing preeclampsia early in pregnancy comes from NICE (National Institute for Health and Care Excellence). NICE is one of the main sources for clinical guidance in the UK along with the RCOG.

Aspirin prophylaxis is recommended if one of the following criteria applies to you: A previous pregnancy with pregnancy induced high blood pressure or pre-eclampsia, high blood pressure outside of pregnancy, Diabetes, chronic kidney disease or lupus.

If you have two of these factors, you will also be advised to take aspirin: It's your first baby, you are 40 or older, your last baby is over ten years old, you have a body mass index of over 35, you have a close relative who had preeclampsia, you are carrying more than one baby (RCOG 2015).

Aspirin is most effective when started before 16 weeks of pregnancy. NICE guidelines on hypertension in pregnancy (2019) recommend taking it until the birth of your baby or until a diagnosis of preeclampsia. Usually your care providers will prescribe it at the booking appointment if you meet the criteria and if your health and social care trust have implemented the policy.

Let's take a look at what evidence there is on prophylactic Aspirin in pregnancy. NICE don't specifically cross reference the evidence they used to support their guidance (or at least I couldn't find any cross-reference), however the ACOG (American College of Obstetricians and Gynaecologists) references various randomised controlled trials (RCT), a meta analysis of 31 RCT, a Cochrane review outlining a meta analysis of data from 59 RCT in their guidance, all of which found that low dose aspirin is moderately effective at reducing the rate of pre eclampsia in women with risk factors (ACOG, 2019).

By exactly how much your absolute risk reduces if you take low dose aspirin in pregnancy is hard to quantify. The ACOG (2019) suggests that your reduction in absolute risk depends on your baseline risk of developing pre-eclampsia in the first place and that is also hard to quantify.

In order to get an idea of what this might mean in real life numbers, I went to look at data from an RCT published in 2017 studying the effects of aspirin versus placebo in 1776 women at risk of developing preterm preeclampsia, meaning the risk of developing preeclampsia before 37 weeks (Rolnik., et al, 2017). Here is the data:

Outcome	Aspirin Group 798	Placebo Group 822
Preterm preeclampsia	13 (1.6%)	35 (4.3%)

This means that aspirin prophylaxis can potentially prevent 27/1000 cases of preterm preeclampsia according to the data from this study. There was no difference in the incidence of preeclampsia after 37 weeks.

Are there any downsides to this intervention?

Aspirin is one of the most commonly used medicines in the world and it is generally considered to be safe. It can cause an allergic reaction if you are someone who is sensitive to its active ingredient salicylic acid. It is also in the family of drugs (NSAIDs) that can give you stomach ulcers or make existing ulcers worse. Rare side effects of aspirin include asthma attacks and more common listed side effects include haemorrhage (BNF, 2022). According to the NHS (2021) the side effects of 'mild indigestion' and 'bleeding more easily than normal' (haemorrhage) occur in more than 1 per 100 people using low dose aspirin. If this is a concern to you, discuss this with your prescribing doctor to help you decide if you want to take low dose aspirin in your pregnancy.

What about the effects of aspirin on your pregnancy?

One Swedish study published in 2020 looked at 313,624 women giving birth, 4088 of whom took low dose aspirin during pregnancy (Hastie, et all, 2020) . There was no higher risk of bleeding during pregnancy in the women who took aspirin, however, the risk of bleeding during birth (intrapartum bleeding) was increased in the group of women who did take aspirin (2.9% aspirin users vs 1.5% nonusers). The risk of bleeding heavily after birth (postpartum haemorrhage) was also increased in the group of women who took aspirin (10.2% vs 7.8%), this risk was present after a natural birth but not at a caesarean section. Finally, the risk of babies having a bleed in the brain tissue (neonatal intracranial haemorrhage) was increased in the group of babies whose mothers took aspirin (0.07% vs 0.01%). The risk of a baby having a bleed like this is overall very low as you can see (0.01%). This means that we can't be sure if the aspirin was the cause of the increase in the amount of babies having this complication (0.07%). When something happens so infrequently you would have to study a larger number of women to determine if the intervention is the actual cause of the complication. In this case all we can say is that aspirin may cause an increased risk of intracranial bleeding, however the potential benefit of avoiding severe preeclampsia to your baby probably outweighs this small risk.

So, this is another situation where you have to feel out where you stand on all of this and look at YOUR big picture.

If you have significant risk factors for pre-eclampsia, you could look at lifestyle interventions for high blood pressure in general. There is evidence to suggest that diets high in fibre like a whole food plant based diet for instance have protective effects for pre-eclampsia and diabetes in pregnancy, too (Pistollato, et al., 2015). Whether you decide to go ahead with aspirin or not, making healthy choices now can only be beneficial for you and your little one.

Are you at an increased risk of developing diabetes in pregnancy?

Your pancreas produces a hormone (insulin) which controls the level of glucose in your blood. Some women do not produce enough insulin during their pregnancies and the blood glucose level can rise above normal.

When this happens in pregnancy it is called Gestational Diabetes Mellitus (GDM).

A glucose tolerance test (GTT) is offered to you in order to find out if you have GDM.

GTT is routinely offered to you if any of the following apply to you:

- BMI above 30 kg/m2

- previous big baby weighing 4.5 kg or more

- previous gestational diabetes

- family history of diabetes (first-degree relative with diabetes)

- an ethnicity with a high prevalence of diabetes.

(NICE Guidelines - 2022)

Interestingly GDM is diagnosed in different ways depending on where you are based. Practices even vary within countries (Gestational Diabetes UK, 2022).

Generally you will be asked to fast from 10pm the night before your GTT. In the morning you will be given a certain amount of glucose to drink.

The World Health Organisation recommends a drink called Rapilose℠. It contains exactly 75g of glucose.

Your blood sugar levels are tested before you drink the glucose, followed by one and two hours after drinking the glucose (some providers take only one further blood test).

Your diagnosis of GDM depends on your blood sugar levels at each stage of the test Gestational Diabetes UK, 2022).

Considerations to help you decide if you want to be screened for GDM:

Very often you will be presented with the risks of GDM as a reason to have the test. There is however a bigger picture to consider before you decide.

The rationale for routine screening for GDM:

- Uncontrolled blood sugar levels increase your baby's risk of stillbirth.

- GDM makes your baby larger than average if we don't treat it. Larger babies have a higher risk of a complication called shoulder dystocia particularly with GDM therefore we need to know if you have GDM so we can prevent this and other risks to your baby.

Treatments:

Daily blood sugar monitoring - depending on the results:

- Diet controlled - diet and exercise

- Oral medicine - metformin

- Insulin injections

Potential impact of a GDM diagnosis on your pregnancy:

- Increased anxiety

- More scanning and monitoring

- Early induction of labour

Does finding out improve overall outcomes?

The aim of GDM monitoring is to have fewer babies who have shoulder dystocia and to have fewer babies whose blood sugars fall very low after they are born. This can happen because in an untreated diabetes the baby is used to higher blood sugars and they experience a sudden drop in blood sugars once they are born. This can be problematic for a newborn baby.

Screening for GDM is also aimed at reducing the amount of women who have uncontrolled blood sugars leading to miscarriage, increased incidence of neural tube defects and stillbirth. There is no consensus that any intervention achieves this.

Dr Christopher Hergerty offers a detailed discussion of the wider considerations around routine screening for GDM. A positive diagnosis will drastically change the pregnancy experience in itself. Dr Hergerty offers for consideration that a diagnosis of GDM will likely induce more anxiety, more hospital visits, more screening and generally leads to induction of labour. Women may also perceive their health in an unfavourable way and may be introduced to oral or injectable drugs in order to control the blood sugar. Dr Hergerty reviewed the data gathered in two major trials comparing treatment for GDM to diet and movement interventions alone. He summarises the potential benefits of GDM treatment as follows:

·   an average birth weight reduction of 110 g

·   for every 48 women treated one fewer baby will have shoulder dystocia manoeuvres at birth (but no difference in harm to babies), and

·   reduced hypertension (high blood pressure) (Hegerty, 2019)

Shoulder dystocia manoeuvres are carried out if the baby's head is born and the baby's body doesn't follow easily because the shoulders are caught in the bony pelvis (shoulder dystocia). Shoulder dystocia occurs in about 1 in 150 births (RCOG, 2012) and it is more commonly observed in babies whose mothers are diagnosed with GDM. The rate for diabetics is estimated to be 1.9% (Hansen, et al., 2014), that's around 3 babies in 150 births, so about three times higher.

So in return for having the diagnosis of GDM and the interventions that come with it, including early induction of labour, you potentially get a baby who is on average just over 3 ounces smaller than what they would have been. There is no overall benefit to the baby, however it is associated with fewer occasions where babies receive manoeuvres for shoulder dystocia. Dr Hergerty states: 'Neither insulin, oral hypoglycaemics (drugs that reduce your blood sugar), nor intense glucose control is shown to improve outcomes compared with diet and exercise alone'. In other words, generally adapting a healthy lifestyle is just as beneficial as going down the route of pharmaceutical blood sugar control.

Dr Hegerty offers some interesting viewpoints on the potential long term disadvantages of reducing a baby's predetermined weight. He suggests that the bigger birthweight could have been reflective of the baby's optimal growth in a favourable nutritional environment and that restricting this could have the same disadvantages growth restriction has on babies on the small scale of the spectrum. Optimal growth is considered to reduce the likelihood of cerebral palsy, improve a baby's childhood intelligence and reduce a baby's chances of developing metabolic conditions later in life. This is an interesting angle to take and worth exploring. I have referenced his article in the reference list and provided a quick link to it in the bonus materials.

Dr Rachel Reed gives an amazing account of the wider considerations around GDM and GDM screening for you and your baby in the Midwives' Cauldron Podcast. There are two episodes available in season two of the podcast. Check out the links to the podcasts in the bonus materials.

Again, there is no right or wrong answer when it comes to deciding whether you want to avail of GDM testing. There is good reason to assume that simply adapting a healthy diet and incorporating regular movement in pregnancy offers you a level of protection against developing gestational diabetes.

Please note that these considerations concern GDM and decision making around GDM screening only and do not apply to entering pregnancy with any type of pre-existing diabetes.

Are you at an increased risk of developing anaemia in pregnancy?

At your booking appointment, and again at 28 weeks, you will be offered a FBC (full blood count). A full blood count looks at all the cells that make up your blood and how the blood is composed. The results are estimated in grams of cells per litre of blood (g/l). Haemoglobin is a protein found inside red blood cells and red blood cells are needed to carry oxygen from your lungs around our body and carry carbon dioxide back to your lungs for you to exhale. A low haemoglobin level is called anaemia. If your haemoglobin is low your red cells are also low and that's why one of the symptoms of anaemia is tiredness. Iron helps your body make haemoglobin. So therefore a lack of available iron in your blood leads to a lack of haemoglobin which in turn leads to a lack of red cells. If your levels are relatively low at the start of pregnancy or have dropped significantly in the third trimester you will be advised to take an iron supplement.

Apart from tiredness, anaemia might also make you feel weaker than usual and develop a shortness of breath. You'll be paler than usual due to the lack of red cells. A good way to check for anaemia is to gently pull your lower eyelid down. Look at the colour of the inside layer of tissue. It should be pink. A white colour is a sign of anaemia.

In your first trimester of pregnancy, your haemoglobin levels should be above 110 g/l and 105g/l in late pregnancy, lower haemoglobin levels are associated with an increased risk of bleeding after giving birth and therefore a homebirth or a freestanding MLU birth will not be advised if your levels drop below these values. After the birth of your baby, a haemoglobin level of less than 100 g/l is considered anaemia (RCOG, 2015).

A drop in your level of red blood cells in later pregnancy is a normal physiological process because you are supplying your baby with iron and your blood volume is expanding as your baby and your baby's placenta get bigger. It is a good idea to be proactive through pregnancy to up your intake of nutritional iron as your daily iron demands increase from around 15 mg per day before pregnancy and in the first trimester to around 30 mg per day in late pregnancy (Dr. Martinez-Biarge, 2022). If you have a good varied diet consuming plenty of iron rich foods and you are not tired, short of breath or feeling generally weak you know you are getting enough iron.

There are lots of ways in which you can amp up your nutritional iron. Pulses, greens, seeds and grains, molasses (licorice), tofu and beetroot are just a few examples in which you can up your iron intake. Iron competes with calcium for absorption and likes vitamin C to aid absorption. So combining pulses with tomatoes in your recipes is a good iron boosting combo, be creative! If supplementing is your way forward, take your supplement on an empty tummy with some orange juice and if you are taking a calcium supplement, take it at a different time if possible. Also, avoid caffeinated tea or coffee around the time of taking your iron supplement because caffeine hinders iron absorption (Pavord, et al., 2020)

The most common side effect of iron supplementation is a sore stomach and constipation (BNF, 2022). Some women find the high dose ferrous fumarate or ferrous sulphate tablets difficult to tolerate which is why you may want to be proactive right from the start of pregnancy to avoid anaemia in the first place. Supplementing with more natural herbal preparations rather than with high doses of ferrous fumarate or ferrous sulphate can be easier to tolerate and can build up your red cell count over time. This type of supplement is particularly well suited if you are entering pregnancy with haemoglobin levels on the lower side of normal.

Is your baby at risk of being growth restricted?

Growth restriction means that your baby is not growing optimally due to being undersupplied with nutrients. Those babies will be smaller than expected for the completed pregnancy weeks. This is described as small for gestational age and can be due to 'intrauterine growth restriction' (IUGR). IUGR is a risk factor for stillbirth.

If your baby is considered to be at risk of being growth restricted, you will be offered a referral for serial scans from around 29 weeks. This is assessed via a screening tool taking into consideration your age, lifestyle habits like smoking, drug use, your dietary habits and fibre intake. Whether you have had a small baby before, if you have had a stillborn baby before, any pre-existing high blood pressure or diabetes and your wider medical history are also considered. If your body mass index makes it difficult for a midwife to measure your bump by doing a symphysiofundal height measurement or if you have fibroids which would also distort findings from the tape measurement you'll also be offered a referral for serial growth scans (RCOG, 2014). Usually scans are performed by an obstetrician at intervals that depend on your history and on what the findings are at each scan.

Symphysiofundal height measurements and customised growth charts

If you don't have any risk factors, your midwife will offer to monitor the growth of your baby bump with a measuring tape and plot the measurement on a customised growth chart.

Here's what you need to know to make an informed decision about whether you would like to have your belly measurement plotted on a growth chart in a 'low risk' pregnancy:

The practice to routinely monitor all babies' growth by using a customised growth chart is a practice that was introduced to identify 'small' babies. A low birthweight is associated with higher morbidity (likelihood of being ill at birth) and a higher risk of being stillborn. A cohort study published in 2013 that evaluated births that occurred between 2009 and 2011 in 19 maternity units in the West Midlands found that the overall stillbirth rate per 1000 births was 4.2. When growth restriction was detected, the stillbirth rate rose to 9.7 per 1000 births and when a baby's growth restriction was not detected the stillbirth rate was increased further to 19.7 per 1000 births (Gardosi J, et al., 2013). You can see that a growth restriction significantly impacts your baby and how finding a growth restricted baby is a good thing that can reduce your baby's risk of being stillborn.

Customised growth charts were introduced as part of a care bundle called the 'Saving Babies' Lives Care Bundle' (NHS England, 2019) along with an impetus to tackle smoking in pregnancy, raising awareness about observing your baby's movements, seeking to improve the ability to monitor your baby's heartbeat in labour and reducing the amount of preterm births. A link to the Saving Babies' Lives v.2 care bundle is available in the bonus materials for you and referenced in the reference list. Staff are trained in how to use growth charts according to the Growth Assessment Protocol (GAP) introduced into practice by the Perinatal Institute for Maternal and Child Health (Perinatal Institute, 2020).

A customised growth chart assumes that women have similar sized babies based on their height, weight, ethnicity and any babies they have already had. Many health and social care trusts use a software called GROW (Hugh et al., 2021), and the health and social care trusts pay this company money every year for the licence. I use this software frequently myself at booking appointments. The software allows your midwife to type in all your data and then it produces a printout with a graph and three lines on it. There is a line that gives you the smallest normal size of a baby for your height, weight and ethnicity and another line for the biggest normal size. Those two lines represent the 10th and 90th percentiles as calculated by the software. The fainter line in the middle is the 50th centile - assumed to be the bang on average size for your baby.

A ten year evaluation of all births in England and Wales between 2008 and 2017 found that those units who applied all aspects of the GAP program were able to reduce their stillbirth rates the most. The study included over 6.5 million births for evaluation. During the ten years that data was collected for, there was an overall decline in stillbirth in all units. By 2017, the still-birth rate in the units that had not implemented the GAP program dropped from 5.12/1000 to 4.37/1000, while that in the units with complete implementation of GAP dropped further, from 5.06/1000 to 3.99/1000 (Hugh et al., 2021).

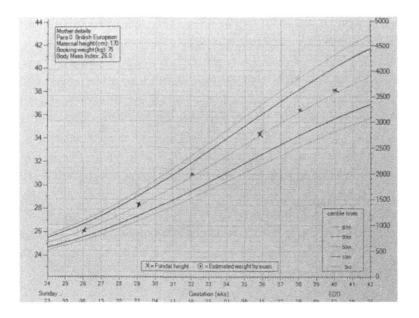

One of my clients kindly allowed me to take this picture of her growth chart. This is an example of a chart with measurements along the 50th centile, no indication to refer for a scan at all.

Like any other screening tool Growth Charts have their limitations and like any other intervention they will inevitably lead to more intervention in women who may not need them.

I find that women feel reassured by this type of chart, however, not all charts require no further investigation. In my experience the chart is very sensitive to measuring irregularities during the first measurements at around 26 weeks when around five millimetres on the measuring tape will make the difference between plotting on the 10th and 90th centile.

If your midwife's measurement puts your baby below the 10th centile you will be referred for an ultrasound scan. The same goes for a sudden increase or a sudden or slow decrease over time in the plotted curve. In my experience it is very likely that you will be referred for a scan if your bump was measured at 26 weeks due to this small margin at the start. This is a consideration if you are keen to avoid ultrasound scans.

There's also the question if the growth chart alone offers any benefit to your baby. Any intervention that is introduced as part of a bundle brings with it the difficulty of determining which part of the bundle brings the benefit. It is also worth considering that estimating your baby's size brings with it the potential for further interventions such as being offered an induction of labour because your baby is thought to be small or big.

According to a study published in 2020 in a professional journal called Ultrasound in Obstetrics and Gynaecology that looked at 11 million births, there is no conclusive evidence to suggest that customised growth charts improve babies' outcomes (Iliodromity, et al., 2020).

If your baby is small because of an actual problem then this is a true hazard for your baby. As we have seen earlier this increases your baby's risk of stillbirth and an induction of labour or a planned caesarean birth may be best for your baby in those circumstances. The question is whether growth charts offer your baby an advantage in and of themselves in return for the potential of introducing interventions for a baby who is absolutely fine. Despite the fact that overall babies' risk of stillbirth has declined in recent years, the answer is that we simply don't have evidence to suggest that it is because of using growth charts for low risk mothers. It will be difficult to ever establish this data because the charts were introduced as part of a bundle and therefore there are other variables to consider, like the fact that lifestyle interventions such as smoking cessation clinics were introduced at the same time (Iliodromity, et al., 2020).

In summary, growth charts are a screening tool for finding babies who are growth restricted when women don't have risk factors that indicate serial growth scans. They were introduced as a care bundle and there is evidence to suggest that those units who implemented the entire GAP program were more successful at reducing the rate of stillbirth than those units who didn't. On the flip side, measuring tapes and growth charts are not an entirely benign intervention. They can lead to a referral for ultrasound scanning in a low risk pregnancy which can lead to a cascade of further intervention when it may not be needed. Ultrasound scans in themselves have a margin of error. If you were referred for a scan at all, it is common to be advised to have a further scan to confirm that the baby is plotting along the same centile in subsequent scans. In my experience scans and the findings during scans have the potential to introduce anxiety in an otherwise normal pregnancy particularly if you are planning a physiological labour and birth. It is common practice to offer an induction of labour for a 'big' baby as well as for the baby who is thought to be small. If a baby is truly growth restricted, finding that baby can significantly improve the potential outcome for this particular baby.

Like with any other screening tool it is good to be clear on what you would do if the result indicated further investigations. How would you feel if a scan was suggested? How would you feel if the scan found your baby to be 'big' or 'small'? Would you feel very anxious in between appointments? How would you decide if you were offered an induction of labour before your due date? How much would normal measurements reassure you? Would normal SFH or ultrasound findings reduce your anxiety? How would you feel if no attempt was made from a professional to monitor your baby's growth? Are you confident in your body and are you actively taking responsibility for your lifestyle choices? Where do you put your trust; do you trust yourself over modern medicine or is it the other way around? Would you feel confident tapping into your own ways of knowing that your bump is growing? Would you feel more reassured if your midwife measured your bump?

In order to decide if you would like a growth chart used in an otherwise normal pregnancy, evaluate your own big picture and weigh up the data against your values, beliefs and your intuition and instinct. It is important to know that you can opt in or out of any aspect of your care and that you can change your mind, too, if you would like to change course.

Have you had a caesarean section before?

If you have had a caesarean birth before, It is now common practice to offer you a vaginal birth after a caesarean section (VBAC) if you want it. If you would prefer another caesarean birth, your choice will also be facilitated.

Generally a vaginal birth is associated with fewer complications than a caesarean section. The benefits of having a physiological birth include a shorter recovery time, you are more likely to have skin to skin contact with your baby immediately at the birth, your hospital stay will be shorter and your baby is less likely to have breathing problems . You are also more likely to have a vaginal birth in any future pregnancies (RCOG, 2016).

When you have had a caesarean before, the scar on your uterus can break. This is called a uterine rupture. A uterine rupture can happen whether you have a VBAC or a planned repeat caesarean birth, it is however more likely in a VBAC. To put it into perspective, your risk of a scar rupture for VBAC is 1:200 versus 1:5000 with a planned caesarean birth (RCOG, 2015). A uterine rupture is a dangerous situation and can be fatal for you and your baby, however the risk of dying during a VBAC for your baby is comparable to that of a first time mother (RCOG, 2015). For you VBAC is safer. Your risk of dying during a VBAC is 4/10000 versus 13/10000 with a planned repeat caesarean birth.

Overall, your chances of having a caesarean section if you go into labour spontaneously after having had a previous caesarean are about the same as those of a first time mum. After one previous caesarean section about 3 out of every 4 women will have a vaginal birth and one woman will have a caesarean section. When you have had a vaginal birth before, your chances of having a VBAC are 80 - 90% (RCOG, 2016).

VBAC is generally advised to happen in a maternity hospital and continuous monitoring with a CTG machine is routine protocol. It is worth knowing that your chances of having a VBAC vary from care provider to care provider along with their overall caesarean section rate. It would be worth checking if there is a special clinic focusing on VBAC and what the VBAC success rate is before making your decision of where you will give birth. It is also worth noting that out of guideline care for VBAC at home can be requested. Your care team will explore your big picture with you and see if there are factors other than the previous caesarean to consider. You'll then be able to make a decision considering your personal big picture.

Urine screening and the other blood tests

Screening your urine for urinary tract infections (UTI) in pregnancy is based on the rationale that pregnancy leaves you more prone to UTIs and that UTI can increase your risk of preterm labour and early and late miscarriage (Public Health England, 2019). A sample of your urine is sent at booking and if there is evidence of infection, you will be offered a course of antibiotics to treat the infection.

There are some simple ways in which you can be proactive about avoiding UTIs in the first place. You can increase your intake of fluids, specifically water throughout your pregnancy to prevent a UTI from developing in the first place. At the risk of stating the obvious: wipe front to back after passing urine in order to avoid bacterial contamination around your urethra. My granny used to treat UTIs with chamomile tea in the years before access to antibiotics and that's what I still use to this day if I feel that a UTI is in the early stages of developing. I have personally not used an antibiotic for many years in any context of my health and this is because I consume very little to no processed sugar and because I am proactive about observing my body for early signs of an issue developing. I usually respond by resting and supporting the healing that my body is initiating in various ways.

Symptoms of a UTI include a stingy sensation and/or pain when peeing, having to pee frequently, cloudy pee, feeling shivery and feverish, pain across your low back area (Public Health England, 2019). If those types of symptoms persist, become worse or go along with shivering and a fever and back pain right from the start, please contact your care provider, it is likely that upping your fluid intake alone will not be enough.

If your urine has group B streptococcus GBS in it you will be informed of this and you will be offered antibiotics to treat the GBS there and then (RCOG, 2017) . You will also be offered IV antibiotics in labour. This is to minimise the risk of your baby becoming infected with GBS (RCOG, 2017). Neonatal GBS infection is potentially life threatening for a baby and Dr Sara Wickham has written an excellent book outlining the possible benefits and the possible disadvantages of routine antibiotic prophylaxis in labour for women who have had GBS in their urine or in a vaginal swab during pregnancy and who are otherwise deemed 'low risk'. The considerations involve looking at the possible impact for your baby of receiving antibiotics via the placenta versus the potential benefits of preventing early onset neonatal GBS. This, again is a complex topic and your decision will be based on evaluating your bigger picture. What I will say at this stage is that the equation isn't as simple as saying that intravenous antibiotics in labour will prevent all neonatal infection with GBS and that there's a bigger picture to consider. I have referenced Dr Wickham's book Group B Strep explained in the reference list for you and I highly recommend reading it if you have been told that you have GBS this pregnancy.

The other blood tests

Screening for HIV, Rubella, Syphilis, Hepatitis B assessing your blood group and screening for atypical antibodies is available to you at booking.

Routine infection screening is mainly aimed at protecting your baby from cross infection by offering you treatment during pregnancy and in the case of HIV in the early postnatal period. It is entirely up to your discretion to have them.

Are you rhesus negative?

There are four blood types - A, B, AB and O. Your rhesus factor is defined by whether or not your red blood cells have a certain type of protein (the D-antigen) attached to them. If they have it, you are rhesus positive and if you don't, then you are rhesus negative.

If a rhesus negative person receives rhesus positive blood in any context they will make anti-D-antibodies.

This is relevant for a rhesus negative mum who carries a rhesus positive baby. If some of your baby's blood were to enter your bloodstream then you would make anti-D-antibodies. This is called rhesus iso-immunisation.

It is rare for your bloods to mix normally in pregnancy unless there is a 'sensitising event'. A sensitising event could be caused by trauma to your belly, a car crash or a fall for instance. Apart from birth any other sensitising events have to do with interventions such as turning a breech baby head down during an 'external cephalic version' or some invasive genetic tests. There is a chance that some bleeding occurs at the placenta and some of your baby's blood could enter your bloodstream. If you form antibodies in pregnancy, those can cross the placenta and damage the baby's red blood cells. This is called rhesus disease and rhesus disease is a potentially serious complication for your baby. Another occasion where bloods possibly can mix is at birth when the placenta separates. Any antibodies you would make would affect any future babies, not the baby just born.

Rhesus disease doesn't usually affect first babies. It also wouldn't affect a rhesus negative baby, ever. So, if you and your baby's father are both rhesus negative, then this can't happen. Rhesus disease can only affect rhesus positive babies of rhesus negative mothers if isoimmunisation occurred. Before Anti-D 16% of babies of rhesus negative women got haemolytic disease of the foetus and newborn because of isoimmunisation. This dropped to 2% of babies when anti-D started to routinely be given after the birth of a rhesus positive baby in a rhesus negative mum. With the introduction of offering all rhesus negative women anti-D in pregnancy, this dropped further to 0·17 to 0·28%. With this reduction in cases, the chances of a baby dying from haemolytic disease due to isoimmunisation dropped from 46/100 000 births when anti-D was given after the birth only to 1·6/100 000 births with the introduction of anti-D prophylaxis in pregnancy (Qureshi et al., 2014).

Anti-D is offered to all pregnant women who are rhesus negative (NICE, 2008), even though a rhesus negative baby wouldn't be affected by rhesus isoimmunisation. Prophylaxis involves an injection of human anti-D immunoglobulin at around 28 weeks. The anti-D injection prevents you from making antibodies in pregnancy. It is offered again after birth if your baby's blood group is rhesus positive to protect future siblings (NICE, 2008).

The British National Formulary (BNF) is a pharmaceutical reference book that lists all medicines in use in the National Health Service in the UK. It lists two products for human anti-D immunoglobulin, D-Gam and Rhophylac. The listed side effects for human anti-D injections are 'chills, fever; headache; malaise; skin reactions' (uncommon), 'Arthralgia [nerve pain in your joints]; dyspnoea [difficulty breathing]; hypersensitivity [allergic reaction]; hypotension [low blood pressure]; nausea; tachycardia [fast heartbeat]; vomiting' (rare or very rare) and 'intravascular haemolysis [the rupturing of red blood cells]' (frequency unknown). Apart from this it is worth knowing that human anti-D is made from blood plasma and therefore it carries with it the same risks any type of blood transfusion would bring. Namely, there is a small chance of cross contamination with any undetected pathogens. According to the British Committee for Standards in Haematology the likelihood of an adverse event in relation to cross contamination is 1 in 80 000 doses (Qureshi et al., 2014).

Donors are screened for blood borne pathogens and according to the manufacturer's leaflet for both human anti-D immunoglobulin preparations listed in the BNF, donated blood plasma is screened negative for hepatitis A, B and C (HAV, HBV, HCV), HIV and human parvovirus (B19V) using a nucleic acid test (CSL Behring, 2021; Bio Products Laboratory Limited, 2022). The plasma then also undergoes a solvent/detergent treatment (using tri-n-butyl phosphate and Triton™ X-100) that is 'effective in inactivating enveloped viruses such as HIV, HCV, and HBV'. The blood plasma is then filtered using a filter 'validated to be effective in removing both enveloped and non-enveloped viruses'. After the solvent treatment and filtering process the excipients of glycine and sodium chloride are added to the human plasma (CSL Behring, 2021).

Some women are like to avoid medicines in general and particularly injectable drugs. Most people would like to avoid injections they don't need and in the case of anti-D there is one scenario that will definitely tell you that the prophylaxis would be entirely unnecessary!

If you and your baby's dad are both rhesus negative, your baby will be rhesus negative too and therefore isoimmunisation can't occur. You can ask for your baby's father's blood type to be checked either in the maternity service or privately so you can avoid an unnecessary injection.

If your baby's father is rhesus positive the question of opting in or out of the prophylactic treatment in pregnancy becomes more complex. May I again point you to Dr Wickham's work for a comprehensive and nuanced exploration of the evidence and the bigger picture around anti-D.

On ultrasound scans in general

Ultrasound scanning initially was introduced because it was deemed to be safer for the baby than using x-Ray. At that stage it was still reserved for certain situations only and not suggested for routine use in pregnancy. The Association For The Improvement Of Maternity Services (AIMS) published a booklet in 1994 called 'Ultrasound ? Unsound' that points to some issues around ultrasound scanning that I find are still relevant today. I have linked it in the bonus materials and you can also just type it into your search engine if you are keen to have a look for yourself. Perhaps the most noteworthy part of this publication is a reference to a quote made by Professor Ian Donald in 1980. Professor Donald was a pioneer of the application of ultrasound technology in obstetrics. Forty years after he first became an advocate for its use Professor Donald said this:

'Perhaps the time has now come to stand and stare and to take stock of where we are going…bearing in mind that sonar…must never lose (its) subservice to the medical art and the paramount importance of the patient…Viewed with this sense of proportion sonar comes as a commodity only, though with many uses. Out of control it can be an obsession, a tail that wags the dog…Sonar is not a new medical religion… nor an end in itself. A tool exploited for its own sake is no better than a saw given to a small boy for cutting wood, who must presently look around the house for suitable objects of furniture inviting amputation… the possibility of hazard should be kept under constant review.' (AIMS, 1994; Ultrasound ? Unsound, p2)

The question of whether ultrasound rays are safe for use on very tiny embryos and foetuses inside the womb almost never gets asked by women. We just assume that any equipment used by medical professionals so routinely must be safe.

In reality we don't know if ultrasound scanning or using ultrasound technology in any other context (dopplers and CTG machines for instance) is entirely benign, there simply is no conclusive evidence. This is often the case when a routine intervention was introduced before studying its impact. Concerns around ultrasound safety usually involve the fact that heat is generated by the ultrasound probe and that we don't know what impact this has on the cells of a developing foetus. Beverly Beach and Jean Robinson (1994) raise the question of whether there could be a correlation between ultrasound scanning and dyslexia and point to a study conducted in 1984 that found a higher incidence of dyslexia in children aged 7-12 who were exposed to ultrasound when compared to children who weren't. They rightly point out that the study is not a randomised controlled trial and that it doesn't warrant the conclusion that ultrasound causes dyslexia, however the authors feel that it is worth asking such questions. Those sources are quite old but they let you see that ultrasound historically was not seen to be entirely benign and the questions raised at the time have not been answered in the absence of any trial data. What has changed since the publication of the AIMS booklet is that the amount of scanning that is routinely carried out within the UK maternity system has reduced significantly, at least in theory. Guidelines do not support a scan at each appointment and I have seen the overall use of casual scanning decline during my time as a midwife.

Ultrasound scanning in the UK is regulated by The British Medical Ultrasound Society (BMUS) and BMUS do recognise those gaps in our knowledge, Their key principles for the safe use of ultrasound state that it should only be used for medical diagnosis and by people who are trained in its safe and proper use. BMUS points out that ultrasound has 'potential thermal and mechanical bio-effects'. To minimise those effects the machine should be set appropriately and the time of exposure should be limited. To keep the growing infant's exposure to ultrasound to a minimum, clinicians are expected to use frequencies 'as low as reasonably achievable' (the ALARA principle) when performing an ultrasound scan. BMUS also states that scans in pregnancy should not be carried out for the sole purpose of producing souvenir videos or photographs (BMUS, 2009).

Hospital policy for 'low risk' pregnancies reflect this. They suggest that there should only be two scans in the entire pregnancy (the booking scan around 12 weeks and the anomaly scan at 19 weeks) unless otherwise indicated and only women with risk factors are offered serial growth scans.

You can see that the medical community appreciates that we don't know if ultrasound scanning is entirely without effect on your baby and this is reflected in general guidance, however some women opt out of scanning altogether and that's okay, too, particularly when the overall potential benefit of scanning is also not easily quantifiable.

On the flip side, the approach to routine scanning within the NHS leaves many women disappointed. Enter: private souvenir scanning companies. Many women would like to see their baby on the screen and will pay for a 3D scan for the experience. The women and couples I speak to often feel that this is an opportunity to bond with their unborn baby and they are excited to show me pictures on their phones of the computer generated profiles of their babies.

Going for a private scan also comes with considerations though. In my experience companies may not always have referral pathways for situations that warrant further investigation meaning that you may not be able to speak to your NHS midwives or doctors for days if a private scan brings up a question. As you saw earlier, BMUS (2009) also advises against scanning for souvenir pictures and videos only.

Again, whether or not you opt in or out of ultrasound scanning is entirely your decision. There can be a lot of value in knowing that a particular condition exists in your baby and I have personally been involved in the care of a handful of families where knowing ahead of time meant that babies with major anomalies could receive well planned and timely surgery soon after birth and they would not have survived otherwise. I have also been involved in the care of people whose anxiety was through the roof because of things seen on scans that turned out to be nothing to worry about. And scans in late pregnancy to 'watch your baby's growth' can also be stressful for families particularly when they want to avoid induction of labour.

When I was taught to scan, my mentor said:

'Always remember, once you put that probe on a woman's belly you are committed to what you see (or think you see) on the screen.'

I think this advice serves practitioners as well as parents. Reminding yourself of this before agreeing to each scan is a good idea. Do the potential benefits of looking today outweigh the potential disadvantages?

Choosing a place of birth

One of the most important decisions you will make in pregnancy and one that many parents underestimate is the decision of where to give birth. You can give birth at home, in a midwife led unit (MLU) or in the obstetric hospital.

In secret #2 I have referenced evidence published in The Lancet to speak to the safety of homebirth for babies in particular. This meta-analysis pooled data from all over the world for around 500 000 first time births and found homebirth just as safe for babies as hospital birth (Reitsma, et al, 2019; Hutton, et al, 2019). I also already said that women are overall better off at home when it comes to their likelihood of bleeding very heavily or having very bad tearing. Breastfeeding is also more likely to establish well when a baby is born at home. All of those advantages also apply for birth in a midwife led unit (Brocklehurst, et al, 2011). Most of these benefits can be attributed to the fact that a spontaneous vaginal birth is safest for mothers and babies, so I will outline the birth outcomes in statistics according to the Birthplace UK Cohort Study (Brocklehurst, et al, 2011):

79% of first time mums who started labour at home had a spontaneous vaginal birth compared to 69% of women who started labour in an obstetric unit. 45% of first time mums transferred from home to hospital and they were still at an advantage after that. The caesarean birth rate was 8% for the women who planned a homebirth and the instrumental birth rate was 13% compared to 12% caesarean births and 19% instrumental births when starting labour in the hospital. There were also fewer episiotomies in the homebirth group (17% versus 24%).

For women having a second or subsequent baby it looked even better. The spontaneous vaginal birth rate for the homebirth group was 98% versus 93% in the hospital group of women. The transfer rate for women who have had a baby before was 12%. The Birth Place Cohort Study looked at 64000 mums and babies. The comparison here included birth centres as well as home. Out-of-hospital birth was overall associated with a higher rate of spontaneous vaginal births regardless of whether it was at home or in a midwife-led unit.

It is worth noting that the Birthplace UK study did find the babies of first time mothers at a disadvantage when labour was started at home (but not in a midwife led unit). The risk of a first baby dying or having a serious medical problem when labour was started at home was 9.3 babies per 1000 births (about 1 in every 100 births) whilst the risk for babies whose mothers started to labour at the obstetric led unit or a midwife led unit was 5.3 per 1000 births (about 1 in every 200 births), there was no difference in outcomes for second or subsequent babies across the places of birth (Brocklehurst, et al, 2011).

All of those statistics were done on women who were assessed as being at a 'low risk' of complications. If you are a first time mum wanting a homebirth and you are confused now because one set of data says first babies are just as safe at home as they are anywhere else and another study says that first babies are at a higher risk of a serious problem at home, I feel you. The study that says it's just as safe (The Lancet Study) was powered by almost half a million babies all over the world and the one that found there to be a difference looked at significantly fewer births - about 64 000. Your decision about the data will depend on whether you feel more reassured by the significantly higher amount of data or, if you are based in the UK, you might place more value in the one that was done in the maternity system that's relevant to you and make a decision from there. You might consider how far you are away from a hospital, you might consider the possible long term effects and make your decision from there.

Evaluate your big picture, listen to your gut and go with what feels right to you. Ultimately data is *just* data, every family is unique. Your values and beliefs are unique to you, your journey is yours. Available data is just one factor in your decision making process.

If you are thinking of having a homebirth or a birth in a midwife led unit inform your providers early so that you can find out if you have any risk factors that would lead them to advise you otherwise.

If this is the case, you can still avail of your chosen place of birth, however it will take more communicating and, depending on the set up in your area, you may have to make yourself known to the head of midwifery or the consultant midwife. Generally, appointments with the wider team will be arranged for you where your risk factor(s) and the considerations around it are outlined to you in detail. Women often report feeling that this is a 'fear mongering' exercise, it really isn't meant to be. Stay open to hearing all of the concerns and engage with the data presented to you so that you can use your logic and your instincts to make a final decision. Remember that the outcome measures that are applied within mainstream healthcare are based on your and your baby's physical wellbeing primarily. That's just the way it is and as long as the communication is factual, this conversation can add to your fact finding project and inform your decision. You'll be able to ask questions and you might decide that you do want to change your mind and go to the suggested place of birth, rather than the one you had in mind first. Either way, hopefully you will find the conversation to be constructive and that your decision to step out of guideline if you wish will be supported even if you sense that your providers don't agree with you.

Common reasons to be risked out of homebirth initially:

· Your age

· Your body mass index

· Having had more than 5 babies before

- If you have had a postpartum haemorrhage and needed a blood transfusion before

- A caesarean section

- Assisted conception

- Your waters have released for more than 24 hours

- Any major medical conditions

- If you have had 3rd or 4th degree tearing before

- Current GBS

- If your baby is suspected to have a congenital anomaly

Later in pregnancy:

- If you have GDM

- If your baby's weight is estimated above the 90th centile or below the 10th

- If you go past your estimated due date and you arrive at the point where induction of labour is offered in your area

This list is not extensive and is based on the 'Guideline for admission to midwife-led units in Northern Ireland' (GAIN, 2018) and on my own experience.

Freebirth

Birth outside the system, unattended birth or 'freebirth' has been around for as long as I can think. It simply means that you don't seek out a midwife or obstetrician to help you during birth, you might give birth with your partner or husband, a friend, a radical birthkeeper or all by yourself instead. Some women also choose not to avail of any mainstream maternity appointments at all during pregnancy. I remember a freebirth in an intentional community I used to visit in Germany about 30 years ago. I was in my early 20s and not a midwife yet. I didn't know the family but I remember getting a glimpse at the newborn baby and being totally amazed that someone just did that.

The subject of freebirth has been topical in the UK recently as more and more women have been choosing freebirth, particularly when hospital visiting and birth companionship have been restricted and homebirth provision cancelled in some areas over the last three years. Women of all walks of life have been taking matters into their own hands and experienced birth unmedicated and on nobody's timeline.

Unfortunately I have no evidence to present to you about how choosing a freebirth impacts on 'safety' as defined by mortality and illness related to birth. We know that midwifery care improves outcomes for mothers and babies on a global level (WHO, 2019; Renfrew et al, 2014) but the data to demonstrate this is at least in part collected in low income countries. It is much harder to establish the impact of institutionalised midwifery care in high income countries where midwifery has become embedded in the medical systems for decades. As well as institutionalised midwifery care in high income countries, shelter, clean water and good nutrition are also more easily accessible than in low income countries. There's also usually access to emergency care in high income countries should the need arise. According to Renfrew et al (2014) 94% of all maternal deaths between 2010 and 2017 occurred in low and lower middle-income countries. Renfrew et al (2014) state that the biggest improvement in mothers' outcomes was seen in Sub-Saharan Africa where the maternal mortality rate decreased by 40% since 2000. I think that it is very likely that the intervention there was to train midwives in how to stop a haemorrhage or how to recognise and treat sepsis. These are among the leading reasons for a mother's death globally (Renfrew et. al, 2014) and big improvements can be made by acting on them quickly. The potential impact of accepting midwifery care may not be the same for a woman in a high income country making an informed decision to step away from institutionalised maternity care. What I mean is, we can't assume that a mother's risk of dying increases by 40% because she chooses freebirth. It's much more complex than that.

We also don't have any data on what the difference in outcomes for babies is likely to be when their births are attended by midwives compared to freebirth. In order to get a true reflection of how freebirth impacts your and your baby's physical safety when compared to accessing maternity services in high income countries, we would need to conduct a study comparing the two approaches. To my knowledge, freebirth outcomes have not been quantified like this yet. Instead, there are plenty of opinions available on the matter from midwives, the media and members of the general public who base their estimation of what the impact of freebirth might be on the assumption that parents lack formal training in obstetric emergencies and that birth is generally dangerous. The freebirth community in turn gives numerous accounts of safe arrivals and birth stories which remind us that women's bodies tend to work - in birth and otherwise. They point out that interventions introduce risks that aren't present when birth can unfold undisturbed and that babies can die in hospitals as well as anywhere else.

I have already quoted the latest MBRRACE-UK statistics to you which illustrates that birth is generally safe in the UK. When we consider freebirth, we have to acknowledge that those figures have been produced within the mainstream system of maternity care and that we don't know if and how birthing unattended affects them.

There's a bigger picture here, too. For many women, perceived physical safety alone does not represent overall safety of body, mind and spirit. Women find the technocratic approach to pregnancy and birth is losing sight of the spirituality of birth, they don't find any connection to the deeper spiritual aspects of birth in clinical settings. They also point out that frequent disruptions are counterproductive to the flow of labour and that that in itself could be considered a 'risk'. The modern industrial approach to midwifery and childbirth is often the reason women in high income countries turn away from maternity services (Dahlen, 2020). The fact that women can get damaged by obstetric practices both physically and mentally is often a deciding factor for freebirth families, many of whom have had experience of institutionalised maternity care during a previous pregnancy. 30 000 women per year in the UK report trauma or suffer post traumatic stress in our maternity services (Birth Trauma Association, 2022). Their partners, too, can feel traumatised by their experience of birth and they can feel like a 'spare part' within services rather than a new parent on their own unique journey. And I already mentioned that some families simply chose freebirth because they weren't going to be separated for one of the key experiences in life. They felt that there was an overreach from the system when partners were excluded from birth rooms during parts of the last three years.

Some parents feel that the short term outcome measures applied to define safety in maternity services are neglecting to examine the possible long term effects of modern industrial maternity care on the overall health of our societies. They point to the ever increasing induction of labour rates, the potential impact of the routine prophylactic use of antibiotics around the time of birth and the possible long term effects of institutionalised birth on our relationships with our children and spouses. Birthing outside the system feels like the safest option to some people.

For other people it is just a situation that evolved. They may have accessed parts of care and not others or they may have gone to all their appointments, they may have had midwives on call for a homebirth and either didn't make it on time to call them or made the decision that it felt okay not to.

There are also families who ended up giving birth unattended who would have liked a supportive and compassionate midwife by their side but couldn't find one. People's experiences are nuanced and the accounts of the families are all very different. As a midwife I feel strongly that every family who would like the care of a midwife should have access to one who fully supports their choices. Pressures on midwives within the maternity system and the effects of having to have conversations around guidelines and risk sadly mean that not all families have access to a midwife or find one they feel they can trust (Dahlen, 2021).

There's no one reason for deciding to have a freebirth or one type of family choosing it, it's a colourful mix of stories. It is also not for everyone. Not everyone is prepared to take on all the responsibility themselves, most people would like to outsource some or all of it. Stepping away from maternity care has implications beyond the practical aspects of observing a pregnancy and birth alone. Even though freebirth rates are on the rise, it is still counter cultural and generally associated with stigma and disapproval from many angles. Some midwives still mistakenly believe that the practice is illegal and some freebirthing parents have been referred to social services by maternity care providers. Women can be seen as naive, victims to a trend glorified by pretty images on Instagram and unaware of the real dangers of childbirth. Parents feel the stigma. Having read and listened to many accounts of the decision making process that is involved in freebirth, I think that it is often the freebirthing parents who are most conscious of all possible outcomes of pregnancy and birth. In the stories I have encountered, the decision to step away is carefully considered and it takes a lot of ongoing work on accepting the unknown throughout the pregnancy in the absence of those things we associate with 'knowing' today. Freebirthing parents go through great lengths to prepare for giving birth and in my opinion they are shouldering a lot. This decision isn't made lightly just as much as a decision to have a planned caesarean birth is never made lightly. Trusting your body, your baby and the process of birth to the extent of going it alone sounds like a challenging journey in and of itself. But you also have to trust yourself to recognise if you do need help from the outside and to potentially face the disapproval and judgement from others particularly if something was to go wrong. On the flip side it sounds like an incredibly rewarding journey for the women and families who choose it.

If you are choosing to give birth unattended by a midwife for whatever reason, I highly recommend that you engage with materials specifically about freebirth in order to prepare fully. Sarah Schmid, a German freebirther has provided a great resource in her book 'Freebirth'. Sarah and her husband are both doctors which gives good insight into the medical culture of birth and the counter narrative. Sarah has 9 children now, including a set of twins, and her children, apart from the first baby, were all born unattended by a midwife, sometimes under the trees and sometimes in the four walls of their home. The book includes a variety of stories including when women chose to transfer into hospital.

There's also the Freebirth Society podcast. It is a great resource for listening to birth stories from all over the world. For a UK based podcast on freebirth, I recommend the 'Normal boring freebirth for normal boring people' podcast which has only just popped up. All of those resources are not only helpful if freebirth is on the cards for you but also if, like me, you are curious about birth in all its expressions. None of the resources shy away from talking about baby loss and potentially occurring problems in labour and birth either.

Finally I found a really informative leaflet for families who are considering giving birth unassisted provided by one of the NHS Trusts in England. It acknowledges freebirth as one of your choices and it gives you information on how to register your baby's birth. It outlines what NHS care is available to you at any point in your pregnancy and how to access it should you want to. The leaflet also includes links for accessing further information on the subject from Birthrights and AIMS (Association for the Improvement of Maternity Services) both of which have information on the legal aspects of freebirth in the UK. You are also given information about who to contact if your choice to give birth unassisted is due to feeling a lack of support from your maternity care providers and you really would prefer to have a midwife present, I have linked the leaflet in the reference list as well as the links to Birthrights and AIMS.

Membrane sweeps

A membrane sweep is a vaginal examination. Your midwife or doctor will insert two gloved fingers into your vagina and palpate for the neck of your womb, your cervix. If your cervix is already a little bit open, the practitioner can insert one or two fingers into it and sweep around the baby's membranes, it is common practice to also stretch your cervix at this point. This procedure causes the release of intracervical prostaglandins. It is thought that this results in your labour starting and it is often presented in a way that assumes that this happens a lot.

It is difficult to say how effective a membrane sweep is when compared to not performing it. If you go into labour after a membrane sweep, it is hard to say whether you were going to do the same without it.

The evidence on how effective this technique is is not conclusive. Let's look at the latest Cochrane review on membrane sweeping published in 2020. The review looked at 44 randomised studies that reported on 6940 women and it found that without membrane sweeping 598 per 1000 women went into labour and 723 per 1000 women went into labour with membrane sweeping (Finucane et al, 2020). That's a relatively small difference (approximately six in ten women versus approximately seven in ten women) and there were differences in the timing of the sweeps and how often they were carried out.

The authors themselves conclude the following:

``We found women randomised to membrane sweeping may, on average, be more likely to experience spontaneous onset of labour (low certainty evidence) and may, on average, be less likely to experience an induction of labour (low certainty evidence). However, these findings should be interpreted with caution as on sensitivity analysis, we found no difference between groups for the outcomes of spontaneous onset of labour and induction of labour.'

This means that we can't be sure that a membrane sweep offers you any increase in your chances of going into labour 'spontaneously'.

Membrane sweeps are now offered routinely to everyone at 39 weeks. This is a change suggested by the new NICE guidelines on Induction of Labour issued in November 2021. In the previous 2008 guideline membrane sweeps were to be offered to first time mums at 40 and 41 weeks and to women who have had babies before at 41 weeks. This means that the suggestion of intervention has moved forward by one to two weeks. There's a suggestion here that your body will not start labour unless someone does something.

NICE lists membrane sweeps as a method for inducing labour and that is what they are. A membrane sweep is the first step in a list of procedures leading up to an induction of labour. So if you are going to opt in to an induction of labour, you might feel that you want to also have a membrane sweep. Inductions of labour are now routinely offered at 41 weeks and we talk more about this.

In my experience many practitioners see membrane sweeps as a procedure that can help you go into labour naturally rather than as an intervention. For many years I looked at them as a benign procedure that may or may not be beneficial. Membrane sweeps and inductions of labour have been so normalised that we have forgotten that a physiological labour is one that starts without any intervention. The disadvantages of sweeps are not always highlighted when the idea is presented to you. They are:

· Bleeding (generally minimal) in the 24 to 48 hours after the sweep

· Cramps and discomfort and loss of sleep in the days leading up to labour

· Vaginal examinations are uncomfortable

· A small chance of your waters breaking during the procedure leading to the possibility of having your labour induced sooner than you might otherwise have chosen

· The suggestion that you 'need' external input for your body to function 'properly' can undermine your confidence and trust in yourself

There's a potential risk of introducing infection during any vaginal examination, however the absolute risk of this when compared to doing nothing is difficult to quantify and likely low. The studies included in the Cochrane review compared membrane sweeping with a mock procedure meaning that all the women had a vaginal examination, so there was no control group who didn't have any intervention. It also didn't measure infection as an outcome. Baby admissions to the neonatal unit were not significantly different between the two groups.

If you would like to take a closer look, check out the references or download the bonus materials for quick links to all the evidence quoted.

If your waters release before labour

Very often your baby's bag of waters will release at some stage in labour. This is called spontaneous rupture of membranes (SROM). Sometimes the waters don't release at all and your baby emerges inside the water bag, the baby is born 'en caul'. In times gone by this was associated with a number of different beliefs and it was generally associated with good luck.

Your baby's bag of waters can also release before you go into labour. Usually you will notice a sudden gush of fluid that keeps coming, you can also have a slow trickle of water. If you think your waters have released, contact your care provider and ask for further advice. Here, we will discuss what your options are if this happens around the time of your due date rather than pre-term.

If your waters go before labour, the question will be: Do you want to wait for labour to start on its own or do you want to have your labour induced?

Practice varies around the world but also between care providers in the same country or sometimes even in the same city. You may be asked to come for a check of your and your baby's heart rate, and your temperature because a deviation in either or both can indicate an infection. You'll be asked to describe the colour of the fluid. Usually you'll be wearing a sanitary pad and your midwife might ask to see it. Sometimes the water can have a slight tinge of pink which usually settles. Your water can also have a greenish discolouration and that may indicate that the baby has passed some meconium (the baby's first stool) into the water. Meconium is quite common around 40-42 weeks and your care providers will recommend a path of action according to your overall pregnancy history and their policies and guidelines. Generally clear water is reassuring and any discolouration may need to be observed.

In the UK recommended practice is guided by the NICE guidelines for induction of labour (2021). NICE suggests that if your waters have released and there is no reason for concern, you should be given a choice to induce your labour right away or wait up to 24 hours. The rationale for inducing your labour is that the risk of infection for your baby increases after the waters have released, however NICE recognise that this risk is overall low and that your wishes should be respected should you want to wait and for labour to start on its own for longer than 24 hours (NICE, 2021).

According to the NICE (2017) guidelines for care in labour your baby's risk of serious infection is 1% rather than 0.5% if your waters hadn't released. NICE also states that 60% of women will start to labour within 24 hours after SROM. In her book 'Inducing Labour, Making Informed Decisions, Dr Wickham quotes a study performed in 1997 that found that by 96 hours after having had a SROM, 94% of women will have gone into labour spontaneously (Wickham, 2021).

How the risk of infection to your baby changes after 24 hours is hard to tell because we don't have any conclusive evidence about it. We do know, however, that risk of infection increases after a vaginal examination and the NICE guidelines recommend that care providers should not perform a vaginal examination if you suspect your waters have released and your labour hasn't started (NICE, 2017). If you decide to wait, you will be asked to monitor your own temperature, the colour and smell of the water and your baby's movements, you will also be advised not to have sexual intercourse to minimise the risk of infection to the baby. Ultimately how long you wait is up to you and your decision will be based on your and your baby's pregnancy history, how supportive your care providers are, your values, your intuition and your own observations.

If you have had a positive group B streptococcus test during this pregnancy the NICE guideline suggests that you should be offered immediate induction of labour or a caesarean section (NICE, 2021).

Induction of labour

First let's look at how labour is induced and then let's look at the evidence for one of the most common reasons for induction which is prevention of prolonged pregnancy.

How it works

An induction of labour is a three step process and it can be initiated in various ways.

The steps are:

1. Softening and 'ripening' the cervix

2. Artificially breaking the waters

3. Intravenous oxytocin drip

You may not need to have all of these steps performed in order to go into labour. If your body was already 'thinking about' going into labour in the next day or two, then your labour could start during the ripening step or after your waters have been released.

There are two ways to soften and ripen your cervix, a mechanical way and a pharmaceutical way.

Mechanical inductions

Mechanical inductions of labour are becoming more common and they involve the insertion of a foley catheter into your cervix. A foley catheter is a silicone tube with an inflatable reservoir near the tip of it. Once the catheter is inserted into the cervix the reservoir at the end of the catheter is filled with around 50 ml of sterile water. The water gets pushed into the reservoir via a syringe and in doing so a small balloon forms between the cervix and your baby's head. When you walk around, the pressure from your baby on the balloon dilates the cervix to around 3-4 cm and the balloon slips out. This usually happens within the first 24 hours but can take longer. During this time you will experience early labour type pain which will generally settle once the balloon has slipped through your cervix.

Where you spend the time until the balloon slips out depends on why your induction of labour is performed. If it is for a non-medical reason such as preventing prolonged pregnancy, it is very likely that you can go home until the balloon comes out.

Once the balloon is out, your cervix is open enough to be able to break your waters. This is called artificial rupture of membranes (ARM) and it is step two in the process of inducing your labour mechanically. Occasionally women go into labour just with the balloon in which case no further intervention is needed.

It is common practice to have CTG monitoring done before you have the catheter inserted. This is to check if your baby's heart rate shows a normal pattern before any intervention takes place.

Usually, once the waters are released, you spend some time walking around to see if your surges start without progressing to step three which is to give you a syntocinon drip. Hospital policy differs in how long you are advised to wait. Four hours is commonly the suggested time, however, if you would like to wait longer to see if your labour will establish, ask your provider how they can facilitate this.

In most places, if labour establishes after those two mechanical interventions you still have the option to go to an alongside midwife led unit and use the birth pool if you wish, however, it is important to know that the transfer rate for slow progress in labour tends to be higher than in a spontaneous labour, particularly if this is your first baby.

If you don't go into labour after the ARM you will go to the labour ward for the syntocinon drip to make contractions. If you need the drip, you will have continuous monitoring (CTG) throughout labour.

Pharmaceutical inductions

Pharmaceutical inductions skip the catheter balloon and use a prostaglandin releasing agent that is inserted into your vagina near the cervix. Prostaglandins cause contractions of the uterine muscle. Again, the induction of labour is likely to be performed in steps and the prostaglandin releasing drug is step one, the one that opens your cervix enough to perform an ARM. The disadvantage of using prostaglandins to prepare the neck of your womb rather than the foley catheter is that prostaglandin containing drugs have side potential side effects.

According to the BNF (2022) uncommon side effects are infection in your baby's bag of waters (amniotic cavity infection), temperature (febrile disorders), headache, jaundice in your baby (hyperbilirubinaemia neonatal), low blood pressure (hypotension), itch (pruritus), an inability of your womb to contract (uterine atony) and vaginal burning. 'Uncommon' describes side effects that occur in between 1/1000 and 1/10000 cases. Side effects of unknown frequency are abdominal pain, diarrhoea, a disruption of your blood clotting ability (disseminated intravascular coagulation), swelling in the vagina (genital oedema), nausea; uterine rupture and vomiting (BNF, 2022).

There are also some contra-indication to using a prostaglandin releasing agent in the first place such as heart or lung disease, if your baby is distressed or not head down or if you have had a caesarean section or surgery to your womb before (BNF, 2022).

If you can be offered a prostaglandin and if you agree, the rest of the induction procedure after your cervix has started to open but you haven't established in labour is the same as I described for the mechanical induction process including the potential option of using the birth pool if your labour establishes without using the syntocinon drip.

The decision of what type of induction is offered to you is based on why the induction is suggested in the first place, your overall health and pregnancy history, on how open your cervix is already and on hospital policy.

The bigger picture and the evidence

Inductions of labour happen in around 50% of pregnancies in some hospitals. Logically it cannot be true, that 50% of babies *need* an induction of labour in order to be *safe*. This is purely related to hospital policy.

In the UK, policy is modelled on guidelines issued by the National Institute for Health and Care Excellence (NICE) or by the Royal College of Obstetricians and Gynaecologists (RCOG). Like membrane sweeps, induction of labour policies refer to the newly issued NICE guidelines.

The new guideline was published in November 2021 and it replaces the previous 2008 guideline.

One of the most common reasons for induction of labour is prolonged pregnancy. Other reasons to offer an induction of labour in an otherwise uncomplicated pregnancy include a suspected big baby, gestational diabetes, or if you are over 40 years old.

Let's focus on a prolonged pregnancy.

In 2008 the guideline recommended that if you are enjoying a normal pregnancy, your midwife or doctor speak to you about the possibility of inducing your labour between 41 and 42 weeks at your 38 week appointment. Membrane sweeping was to be offered at 40 weeks and

41 weeks for a first pregnancy and at 41 weeks if you have had babies before. There was an emphasis on awaiting a spontaneous onset of labour. This is because a healthy pregnancy that leads to a spontaneous labour offers you the choice of giving birth outside of the obstetric unit at home or in a midwife led unit and therefore it increases the likelihood of a spontaneous vaginal birth and all the associated benefits that I have listed in the 'choosing a place of birth' section.

The new NICE guideline has subtly shifted how practitioners are meant to talk to women about induction of labour. The idea that you might 'need' your labour induced is to be introduced earlier in pregnancy now, thus normalising a medical approach to your pregnancy.

The guideline recommends that all women should be offered a membrane sweep routinely at 39 weeks and that your midwife or doctor has conversations with you about the risk of continuing with pregnancy beyond 41 weeks in relation to stillbirth. To make their recommendations, NICE conducted a review of fifteen randomised controlled trials conducted between 1975 and 2019. When accumulating the data, the risk of stillbirth at 42 weeks was stated to be about 35/10 000. The risk at 41 weeks was about 4 babies per 10 000 births representing an approximate increase in risk of 31 babies per 10 000 births. These figures are significantly higher than the overall incidence data on stillbirth reported by MBRRACE - UK in 2021. In the UK between 2016 and 2019 the stillbirth rate between 37 and 41 weeks was 1.17/1000 babies (12 babies in 10 000) and 6 babies per 10000 at 42 weeks. Is this due to an increase in inductions of labour?

Is the reduction partly due to different ways of gathering data per week of pregnancy? Is it due to the fact that some of the studies used by NICE are dating back to the 1970s? What is the impact of induction of labour in itself? There's no easy answer.

The Australian midwifery researcher Dr Hanna Dahlen published a study in 2021 that found that while induction rates have tripled between 2001 and 2016 in New South Wales, the stillbirth rate has not reduced.

The study shows that statistically speaking, induction of labour causes more problems in women and their infants than spontaneous onset of labour does.This comes at no surprise to midwives who have known this intuitively and have long been voicing their concern about this trend to perform more and more inductions of labour.

This paper summarised findings that were gathered over 16 years in Australia (2001-2016) and it is called the New South Wales Study. It's a strong study in that it included almost half a million healthy women giving birth between 37 and 41+6 weeks. The interesting detail about this study is that the researchers followed up with the women to be able to gather data in relation to mother and baby's overall health measured in hospital admissions (Dahlen, et al., 2021).

The overall findings suggest that induction of labour leads to more interventions and poorer outcomes for the mother, baby up until young adolescence.

It is important to remember that this is data based on a population of 474,652 women and their children and whilst the findings are incredibly valuable it does not mean that induction of labour is always bad. There are individual scenarios where opting for an induction is YOUR best way forward, however the main take home point is that, increasingly, inductions are done without a medical reason (this happened to 15% of the women in the study) or without good evidence to suggest that it offers any benefits (Dahlen, et al., 2021).

The study found the following disadvantages of an induction of labour for you:

- Increase of epidural or spinal analgesia use

- Higher chance of having a caesarean section

- Higher chance of an instrumental birth

· Higher chance of having an episiotomy

· Higher chance of having a postpartum haemorrhage

The disadvantages for your baby up until the age of 16:

· Higher rates of birth asphyxia (low oxygen during labour)

· Higher rates of resuscitation at birth

· Higher rates of birth injuries

· Higher rates of respiratory issues

· Higher rates of hospital admissions for infection

If you would like to look at the paper for yourself, it is referenced here and I have linked it into the bonus materials.

In it you will see some other trials mentioned that also didn't find reduction in stillbirth if women had inductions of labour.

You will, however, also see two Cochrane Reviews mentioned where there was a reduction in the rate of stillbirth associated with induction of labour. The number of women and babies having an induction of labour to prevent one stillbirth was 426 in one of the reviews and 544 in the other. (Dahlen, et al., 2021; Middleton, et al., 2018; Middleton, et al., 2020).

Cochrane reviews are literature reviews that pool together trials from across the world in order to collate the data and report the findings. They are therefore recognised by the medical community internationally as 'gold standard' evidence.

It is worth noting though that none of the studies in the Cochrane reviews looked at long term health implications of induction of labour for the infants. Dr Dahlen's study is unique in that way and the question of how medicalisation of birth impacts our species as a whole is an interesting one and an important one for the generations that follow us. If you would like to read more about how induction could impact your baby in the longer term and for a thorough discussion of induction of labour overall, I highly recommend reading Dr Wickham's book 'In Your Own Time' as soon as you can in pregnancy. Also check out the podcasts on induction of labour linked in the resource page.

You can see how much information there is and that the outcomes of various studies can contradict each other. When it comes to evaluating any data, be sure to look at the big picture.

Any study, regardless of how well it is designed, how well biases and conflicts of interest are recognised and controlled for and how large it is can only ever give you a population based result. So, in the case of looking at inductions of labour in late pregnancy and evaluating how it impacts stillbirth, one baby could have benefited from the induction and another baby could have been harmed by the induction process itself. That results in 'no difference in outcome' whilst potentially also leaving one family wishing they had had an induction of labour and another family wishing that they hadn't.

Ultimately, regardless of anybody's best estimation, nobody can look into the future and tell you what is going to happen to you and your baby.

This is why it is so important that you ask yourself what your values and beliefs are when it comes to medical intervention? Where is your locus of trust?

None of this is easy because it is so deeply personal and if this is your first child it'll also be the first time in your life where the responsibility of making a decision on behalf of another human is weighing on you. Getting to a place of accepting this responsibility is a journey and it demands being honest with yourself. If you decide to trust a midwife or doctor's recommendation and you look back wishing you hadn't, you will still arrive at a point in your healing where you realise that you have to take responsibility for that decision as much as you would have to take responsibility for your decision not to. In my experience this becomes a lot easier when all your decisions come from a place of honesty and inner knowing.

In other words, trust your intuition, listen to your inner voice and accept the things you can't control.

Parenting is the best self-development course you could ever join!

Here are some examples of some of the other common reasons to offer an induction of labour in women who are otherwise healthy:

Your Baby Is Estimated To Be Big
You are 40 or older
You had an assisted conception

Your waters have released before labour

Also:
Gestational Diabetes
High Blood Pressure
Small baby
Reduced baby movements

If you would like to have an online consultation exploring your big picture, talk through your fears and you want some help understanding all your options, you can get in touch via https://www.essentiallybirth. com/contact-sevensecrets to find out how I can help you.

Early labour

Early labour or the latent phase of labour is defined in the medical model as the time when your cervix thins out and opens up to four centimetres dilated.

For you this is the time of starting to feel some sensations and the time that your oxytocin receptors start to increase and you are making your special labour cocktail of oestrogen, oxytocin and prostaglandin and your baby signals 'let's go'. These sensations can start and stop for a few days and that can make you feel anxious and question yourself. That's normal, use your techniques, tune in to your baby, trust your body.

Your physiology is asking for darkness, quiet, and a sense of safety. If you have made the decision that safety for you means an MLU or hospital, then you will have to leave your home to travel to an assessment unit. This can lead to a release of adrenaline and momentarily stop your contraction surges. You can counteract this by wearing sunglasses (no kidding) and by using earplugs or listening to some of your favourite comfort tunes on your headphones (this can mean upbeat music, whatever makes you feel at ease).

At your assessment unit you may be offered a vaginal examination. It is common practice to offer paracetamol or co codamol at this stage. Paracetamol (Acetaminophen) is known to be a prostaglandin inhibitor and therefore it can theoretically interfere with labour progress. I have often wondered if the benefit of a warm bath, staying mobile, a TENS machine, warm aromatherapy compresses or simple heat packs can be just as beneficial as using paracetamol. And then I learned that paracetamol theoretically has the potential of inhibiting one of your essential ingredients in the labour cocktail of hormones. The 'undercover midwife' may be the first person who got me thinking about paracetamol in this context in her blog post entitled 'Paracetamol and labour'. She speaks of her observations of how paracetamol has become used so commonly in early labour and she wonders if it could be related to experiencing a long latent phase of labour. I have linked this in your bonus materials. The undercover midwife has also brought up the question of whether paracetamol is entirely benign for the baby, again, she discusses this in her blog, go and have a read.

The sensations of early labour allow you to lean into your bodily sensations and get to know your labouring body. At this stage, prioritise resting when you can.

I was asked recently if aspirin prophylaxis can interfere with early labour in the same way as paracetamol might do. The answer is that I don't know and there is no evidence to suggest it because nobody has looked at it yet. Having said that, aspirin is also known as a prostaglandin inhibitor. If you have chosen aspirin prophylaxis it should be enough to simply stop it once you are starting to observe the onset of labour. To me it also seems reasonable to stop it at around 37 weeks because it appears that aspirin does not impact on the incidence of preeclampsia after 37 weeks (Rolnik, et al., 2017). Please bear in mind that this is simply my opinion and I would advise you to speak to your care provider to discuss your pregnancy history before making a decision.

After your early labour assessment, you will either be advised to return home - in that case check out the bonus materials for my top tips of what to do at home - or you will be admitted to the MLU or labour ward.

If you have chosen homebirth, it'll be all about deciding when to call your midwife. In general I usually suggest that once you feel you need support, reassurance or you feel that your labour is moving along on the continuum to more frequent longer lasting surges you contact your on call midwife.

Routine observations in labour, vaginal examinations and the partograph

Routine observations are offered to you at home, in the MLU or in the labour ward.

In order to perform the routine observations of checking your heart rate, temperature and blood pressure at certain intervals your midwife will need to approach and touch you. This can be done discreetly and I have attended many labours where women were able to stay in their zone despite my approaches. The same goes for listening for your baby's heartbeat. However, when we revisit the physiological birth blueprint, we must acknowledge that every time I approach you at all and particularly when I offer to examine you vaginally, I am potentially interfering with your body's processes. If any finding is outside of the normal parameters as defined by our guidelines, your midwife will have to talk to you about this and ask you what your choices are in the context of these findings.

The NICE intrapartum care guideline (2017) suggests the observations be performed at the following intervals: 4 hourly for blood pressure, temperature and vaginal examinations, hourly pulse and listening to baby every 15 minutes (if you don't have any risk factors). Together with the pregnancy risk assessment and observations that I have described to you, this way of observing labour and birth forms the foundation for the data I have presented to you in relation to pregnancy outcomes. We can say that pregnancy and birth are overall safe in the context of this baseline. We have to acknowledge that when we step away from this, we don't have any data. We also have to acknowledge that, in and of itself we simply can't say what the value is of performing each observation on 'low risk' women in labour when compared to doing nothing. We also have never measured the impact performing the observations has on your labour progress.

Whether you opt in or out of observations will depend on whether you think you will find the observations reassuring and therefore you accept the interruptions or not. If they add to your sense of safety, then they might help your oxytocin flow and therefore help your labour progress. If you feel you want to be left alone with your baby and trust your intuition, then it is absolutely fine to decline them. Both ways of looking at it are valid within their own value and belief systems.

I have attended births where women choose to decline any clinical observations at all. I have also looked after women who decide that they only want observations performed when they themselves feel the need to get input from the outside. Generally most women I have looked after are reassured by hearing their baby's heart beat regularly and a lot of women want to know how dilated their cervix is at some point in labour because this is the context in which they have always known labour to be talked about by family and friends. Other women decline all vaginal examinations because they find them too invasive and counterproductive to their labour flow. Again, this is your personal choice.

A recent cochrane review (Moncrieff, et al., 2022) on routine vaginal examinations concluded this:

'We cannot be certain which method for assessing labour progress is most effective or acceptable to women. Further evidence is needed to identify the best way to assess labour progress and how this may affect women's birth experiences.'

CTG monitoring

CTG monitoring is reserved for women with risk factors or for 'low risk' women who develop risk factors in labour (NICE, 2017). CTG monitoring was introduced into labour wards in the 1970s without evidence to support its use. It was introduced in an attempt to reduce the rate of cerebral palsy and babies dying in labour. CTG monitoring has still not been proven to be effective at doing this and instead it has increased the caesarean section rate (Small, et al., 2020).

CTG monitoring is routinely performed when women have Epidurals, when they have a drip of syntocinon to make contractions and when there are risk factors that put the baby at a higher risk of an adverse outcome in labour (NICE, 2017). Small, et al (2020) did a systematic review of 9 randomised controlled trials and 26 non-experimental studies and found no significant statistical difference in babies dying in labour in women who were deemed at a higher risk of complications when using CTG monitoring compared to intermittent auscultation (listening in every 15 minutes). The authors concluded that the review failed to demonstrate benefits in CTG monitoring over intermittent auscultation and that there is an urgent need for a well designed study to establish if CTG monitoring offers any benefit for women with risk factors.

In summary, we know that CTG monitoring offers no benefits to women with no known risk factors and we don't have any conclusive evidence to say that CTG monitoring offers any benefit to your baby if you do have risk factors (Small, et al, 2020). We also know that CTG monitoring increases your chances of having a caesarean section. This is because the baby's heartbeat trace can look abnormal when everything is fine. According to data collated in a Cochrane systematic review performed by Alfirevic Z, (2017) the risk of caesarean section increased from 66/1000 with intermittent auscultation to 108/1000 with continuous monitoring. In this review the authors found that your baby is at a lower risk of having a seizure after birth but the impact of this is unclear. They said this:

'CTG during labour is associated with reduced rates of neonatal seizures, but no clear differences in cerebral palsy, infant mortality or other standard measures of neonatal wellbeing. However, continuous CTG was associated with an increase in caesarean sections and instrumental vaginal births. The challenge is how best to convey these results to women to enable them to make an informed decision without compromising the normality of labour.'

In my experience the question of declining a CTG when there is a risk factor and guidelines would suggest that the CTG monitor should be used most often comes up when women request homebirths out of guidelines. I know of very few scenarios when a CTG was recommended and declined in the context of a hospital birth. When it comes to monitoring your baby's heart rate in labour, midwives report that they often don't feel they could facilitate a fully informed choice. According to a research article from Australia, this was due to time restraints but also due to fear of litigation. Women typically report that the decision of how the baby's heartbeat would be monitored was made by the clinicians (Small, et al., 2022).

I suggest that you find out early what the recommendation is for monitoring your baby in labour so that you can start thinking about what your preference will be. Dr Kirsten Small is a retired specialist obstetrician who has written extensively about CTG monitoring in various contexts. Her blog 'Birth Small Talk' is a fabulous free resource and in it she shares generously about all things CTG and more.

How labour progress is monitored

Labour progress is monitored on a partogram where midwives plot the findings gathered during a vaginal examination along with the other observations performed in labour. Today's partogram and the expected 'normal' labour progress is based on a study performed by Dr Friedman in the 1950s. Dr Friedman observed 500 women, all hospitalised, in labour and he used a graph to plot the women's cervical dilatation against the time they had been in labour. He divided the resulting graph into three stages and found that labour normally lasted 14 hours. This is how the famous 'three stages of labour' were born along with the 500 babies.

They are:

- First stage of labour - 4 cm dilated to fully dilated

- Second stage of labour - fully dilated to giving birth

- Third stage of labour - birth of the placenta

We still use 'Friedman's Curve' to monitor your labour today. If you don't make progress against this graph measured by how far dilated your cervix is, then interventions like breaking your waters or putting up a drip to speed up labour are offered to you.

Your expected progress in the first stage of labour is this:

1 cm every two hours as a first time mum

1 cm every hour if you have had babies before

(NICE, 2017)

The problem with this is that women are not machines and they don't all dilate at the same rate. You could have your cervix assessed and be told you 'are only 1 cm dilated' and have a baby in your arms in an hour flat or you could be told you are 'fully dilated, meaning all of the cervix has melted away from in front of the baby's head but you still don't even feel an urge to push three hours later. These are the two extreme ends of a spectrum that is as variable and as unique as the amount of women in labour at any given time.

Between 1 April 2018 and 31 March 2019, only 54% of all first time mums had a spontaneous vaginal birth in England and Wales. The caesarean birth rate was 23% and the instrumental birth rate for first time mums was also 23% (National Maternity and Perinatal Audit, 2022). For perspective, the Farm midwifery centre in Tennessee, headed by the iconic midwife Ina May Gaskin, have an overall caesarean section rate of below 2% and they support twin and breech birth. They also have the same safety record for infants as the rest of the USA. The women there don't fear birth, they can move freely, there's no prescribed time limit and they are supported along the lines of a more traditional approach to midwifery (Gaskin, 2002). Yes, we do have to consider that this data gathered among a specific group of women is not directly transferable to a UK population, however there is potential for learning from The Farm community and from the midwives there.

I highly recommend reading the classic 'Spiritual Midwifery' by Ina May Gaskin. It is an extraordinary account of birth, community and social history in the USA.

Pain relief in labour

Pain relief in labour can be categorised in two branches. Non-pharmaceutical, where no drugs are used and pharmaceutical where drugs are used as part of your coping strategy for labour. It is important to remember that there is no right or wrong way here. You are only answerable to yourself. You do you!

Generally, there usually is a point in labour when every single woman is challenged and thinks she 'can't do it'. If you generally feel you want to avoid medical pain relief, then plan for this and instruct your birth partner to support you and remind you and help you over the hump. It's also 100% valid to change your mind at any point. So for instance, usually when someone is now convinced that they 'can't do it anymore', after a bit of upping the ante with non - pharma support, maybe a position change, a good back massage, a trip to the toilet (slowly, slowly), things can settle again and you actually have integrated again with your sensations. If this is not the case, then look at your plan B and perhaps you do want to use pharmacological tools. Make space for this as you prepare so that you can feel good about your experience in hindsight. There are endless ways in which to have a baby.

When I ask about women's ideas about pain relief, I get a huge variety of responses .I have heard 'give me every drug under the sun' and I have heard 'I want to avoid all drugs'. It's okay to change your mind both ways!

Here's the toolbox for pain relief:

TENS (transcutaneous electrical nerve stimulation)

Tens is a little machine that produces an electrical stimulus. You stick four pads on your back and you can press a button that sends the stimulus into the pad. You'll feel a pins and needles type sensation where the pads are right next to your spine. TENS works according to the 'gate control theory' suggesting that there are 'gates' in your central nervous system that allow a pain stimulus to reach your brain. The TENS stimulus is positioned so that that sensation reaches your brain and therefore closes the gate for the labour pain. The TENS offers stimulation to your nervous system so your central nervous system is distracted and the sensation of the surges does (Rodriguez, 2005).

TENS has no side effects, you can use it alongside other methods, you can move around freely with it on but you'll have to take it off in the pool or in the shower.

It's excellent to use at home in early labour, you can combine it with other methods and you can use it all the way through.

Squeezing a comb

You simply squeeze a fine toothed comb in your hand. This also works according to the gate control theory, it's cheap, easy to use and obviously you can use it alongside any other form of pain relief. I have many anecdotal accounts of how this helped. I also remember looking after a very young mum in labour who just wanted her mother to squeeze her hand really hard during each surge and that's how she got through. I would also class hip squeezing and massage down either side of the spine with this specific theory.

Mobilising, massage, reflexology and aromatherapy

Easy to do and particularly useful at home or in early labour. Some small studies suggest that women who receive these support measures report lower pain scores and better satisfaction with pain relief when compared to women who didn't. The movement helps with labour progress (Jones, et. al., 2012; Lawrence, et al., 2013). If you are bringing aromatherapy to the hospital, be sure to use an electrical diffuser, because candles are a fire and explosion hazard around the medical gases in the hospital.

Hiring a doula

Doulas are professional birth partners so to speak. You form a relationship so you benefit from having a familiar person throughout pregnancy and you also have an advocate to communicate your choices in labour. If you have a significant other, you are both supported in your experience. When compared to birth companions who don't have any training about birth and birth related topics a doula may improve your chances of a spontaneous birth (Bohren, et al, 2017) but they can also be great support during elective c/s. Many doulas are trained in aromatherapy and other holistic modalities which all help you cope in labour. When choosing a doula consider interviewing a few people. Just like your midwives or doctors and everyone in your field, a doula can also have biases. We all do. Generally doulas will be very good at keeping you on track for an experience free from intervention and the midwives and doctors will be good at presenting to you any factors that would initiate recommending an intervention. To come to a balanced decision, consider both narratives. A doula is there to help you balance the pros and cons of each way forward so you can come to a decision yourself. If you are making choices that you know are off guideline, let your maternity care team know early on so your journey through the system can be organised and happen smoothly.

Hypnobirthing, yoga and visualisation

In my experience, deep breathing is one of the best strategies for staying on top of your labour surges, the calmness you can initiate in your central nervous system aids muscle relaxation. I have seen surprising results with just consciously changing your breathing pattern in labour even without ever practising before. Women who practise regularly report great effects and satisfaction with an applied breathing practice. Yoga is a great way of practising your deep breathing regularly and it keeps your muscles subtle and stretchy, your body balanced and it allows your baby the room to move through your body. Your yoga practice in pregnancy also gives you an opportunity to connect with your baby and visualise the process of giving birth. Yoga, meditation, music and hypnosis techniques may all have a calming effect and provide a distraction from pain and tension (Jones, et al., 2012).

Labour in water

You simply immerse yourself in water in a birth pool, the water in a birth pool is around body temperature. You feel safe and secure in your own space in the pool. Waterbirth or labouring in water reduces the likelihood of going for an epidural (Burns, et al., 2009). Water may shorten labour and is associated with supporting the birth physiology and the buoyancy makes it easy to move and change position (Jones, et al., 2012). You can still use Entonox. Waterbirth is not recommended when you have risk factors, so speak to your providers early if you have risk factors and would like to go into the water. What you decide will depend on your big picture after weighing up the pros and cons for your particular situation.

Entonox – nitrous oxide and oxygen

This is a pharmaceutical form of pain relief. It is a gas that is delivered via tubing and a mouth piece. You simply breathe it in and out during a surge. The good thing is that it only works when you use it and as soon as you stop it, it stops working. It is thought to have no side effects to the baby and it can be used with the birth pool. It focuses you on your breathing. Nitrous oxide can make you nauseous and you might vomit but that usually settles again. The piping can restrict your movement depending on how much reach it has but generally you can still move about freely within a certain range whilst holding the mouthpiece.

Opiates

Diamorphine and morphine are both used in labour. They are both opiates and they get injected under your skin or into your muscle. Opiates help you relax and therefore they can relax your voluntary muscles which can be helpful if you have been holding on a lot. The disadvantage is that it also relaxes your involuntary muscles and as such it can slow down the contraction pattern. It can also make you nauseous and drowsy and it does cross to the baby via the placenta. Rarely the baby's breathing can be affected at birth and the baby may need a drug called

Naloxone to regulate this. The British National Formulary lists breathing problems with opiates as a 'common or very common' side effect for the person receiving it. This means that the incidence is between 1/10 and 1/100. It doesn't list how often babies are affected, it just points to the possibility of this happening (BNF, 2022). I found little data on how many newborn babies receive Naloxone. I found one study that evaluated the introduction of a 'Good Practice' protocol for assisting a newborn baby with breathing difficulties. It found that 1 in 500 infants of mothers who had received an opiate received Naloxone when the new protocol was observed. This study was conducted in 1998 and the protocol is how I learned to assess a baby before considering giving Naloxone (Box & Cochrane, 2007). More commonly a baby can be sleepy at birth and it may interfere with breastfeeding (Jones, et al., 2012). In my experience opiates can be helpful if you find advanced labour very hard to deal with, are open to using pharmaceutical pain relief and would like to avoid an epidural. You can still use the pool two hours after a dose.

Remifentanil

Remifentanil is an opiate that acts quickly and stops acting quickly. You get a cannula sited to administer it directly into your veins. You also get a PCA device (Patent Controlled Analgesia) meaning that you get to press a button when you need the pain relief, i.e. during a surge. When you use remifentanil, you will need nasal prongs with oxygen and stay on a monitor for your blood oxygen saturation. There is the risk of respiratory depression as you can 'forget' to breathe and your care provider will observe you closely. As with other pain relief medication, there is an increased risk for your baby to need a drug (Naloxone) to reverse the effects of the opiate. According to a cochrane review conducted in 2017 (Weibel, et.al.) women tend to be more satisfied with remifentanil when compared to other opiates and less satisfied than with an epidural, however the authors conclude that the overall quality of the evidence is poor and that more studies are needed. Women in the remifentanil group were overall less likely to opt for an epidural than in the control group of women who received intramuscular opiates. None of the studies looked at how often Naloxone was given to newborn babies (Weibel, et al., 2017).

Epidural and spinal anaesthetic

Epidural analgesia is delivered via a cannula that gets inserted into the epidural space next to your spinal cord. The infusion stays in place for the entire labour. The local anaesthetic drugs delivered via this cannula vary depending on protocol but often involve Bupivacaine and Fentanyl. In labour the epidural gets sited in the lumbar spine area and therefore numbs your legs and torso. Epidurals can take away your labour pain completely and you stay alert. Epidurals can also be 'patchy' and they may leave you with breakthrough pain. When it comes to satisfaction with pain relief, women rate epidurals higher than they rate opiates. Anim-Somuah, et al., (2019) state that 735/1000 women report excellent or very good pain relief with an epidural, compared to 500/1000 in the opium group. Epidurals can make you feel itchy, make your blood pressure drop and they can make you feel nauseous. You will also need a catheter sited into your bladder because you won't be able to pee with your epidural in. The Royal College of Anaesthetists list inadequate pain relief, low blood pressure, itch and nausea as a 'very common' side effect, describing an incidence of one in every ten epidurals (RCOA, 2020). Some hospitals offer mobile epidurals meaning you can still walk around using the effect of gravity, if not, you will be bed bound for your entire labour.

You will usually be monitored with a CTG monitor when you have an epidural. Epidurals are linked with an increase in instrumental birth and in some studies they are associated with more caesarean sections, however this could be because Epidurals are often used in long labours or in inductions of labour, meaning that the epidural itself may not be the only contributing factor. In their Cochrane review, Anim-Somuah, et al.,(2019) found epidurals to be associated with a higher rate of instrumental births (from around 10% with opiates to around 14% with epidurals) but there was no increase in caesarean sections between the two study groups.

Side effects of epidurals are mainly related to the time of getting it sited. The epidural needle can puncture the dura when your epidural catheter is inserted. The dura is the connective tissue that protects the spinal cord. When this happens, cerebrospinal fluid leaks causing a severe headache.

This happens in 1 in every 100 to 1 in every 500 epidurals (RCOA, 2019; RCOA, 2020). It may resolve by itself but it may need to be treated with an epidural blood patch, where some of your blood is injected into the space to patch up the puncture of the dura (RCOA, 2019). In around 1 in 1000 epidurals, the needle can cause nerve damage leading to temporary loss of sensation in an area of your body. This usually resolves on its own but in 1 in 23,500 to 50,500 epidurals the nerve damage is permanent. Very rarely, in 1 in 54,500 to 1 in 141,500, the epidural puncture can lead to paraplegia or death.

One of the advantages of an epidural is that it can be used for a caesarean section if you need one in labour. If not, or if you go for a planned caesarean birth, you will most likely be offered a spinal anaesthetic. A spinal is similar to an epidural but the needle is smaller and it is a one off injection rather than a continuous infusion. A spinal has the same associated risks as stated above for epidurals (RCOA, 2020).

This concludes the pain relief section. Most women who give birth in midwife led units or obstetric hospitals use a combination of methods. At homebirhts some women use breathing and meditation techniques alone and others use them in combination with pharmaceuticals. The decision making process is different for every single woman and each choice is valid. We discuss this in great detail in the R.O.A.D. To Birth Hypnobirth classes. You can join the next cohort via https://www. essentiallybirth.com/road-to%20-birth-secrets-readers.

Bladder care

Bladder care means that midwives will measure everything you drink and they measure the amount of urine you pass. They plot it on an input and output chart and if it seems you retain urine, you'll be offered a catheter.

Keeping your bladder empty is important when you consider that your baby's path is right between your bladder and your back passage. A full bladder can be in the way of labour progress. Generally you'll just pee regularly in labour and everything is fine. Sometimes women can't pass urine even though the bladder is full. In this case try some essential peppermint oil in the toilet bowl or drip some onto a bit of toilet tissue and hold it close to your urethra (not onto it!). This can help you pee. If you can't you'll be offered an in-out catheter to empty your bladder. I have linked a video I made about this in the bonus materials.

Siting an in-out catheter is simple but it can introduce infection and cause a UTI. It is also invasive and can knock your flow. This is why I encourage you to either go to the toilet at regular intervals in labour or to allow yourself to pee into a bedpan or onto pads on the floor or even into the birth pool. Visualise this and make it part of your journaling, visualisations and affirmations. Aim to keep your bladder nice and small for your baby to move past.

And no, not drinking anything at all and getting dehydrated isn't the solution either, because that can stall your surges and your labour progress.

Now for the pooping which can happen as your baby moves lower and lower. This is entirely normal, but sometimes women hold back their pushes because they become self aware of the pressure on the back passage and they are afraid and embarrassed to let go. If you think this could be you, work on accepting that there will be poo. The famous hippie midwife Ina May Gaskin once told me that she uses what happened to be our favourite children's book for the poop chat with her pregnant clients. The book is called "The story of the little mole who knew it was none of his business" and it's a story of revenge (and poop). The little mole wakes up one morning, gets out of his little mole hill and a big poop lands on his head. The little mole goes to investigate who did it. Let's just say it's a great book for birth prep and for potty training kiddies.

Artificial rupture of membranes

This is when the midwife uses a hook to release your baby's bag of water. It is usually suggested to you if a 'delay in the first stage of labour' has been observed. The NICE guidelines for routine care of women in labour

(2017) describe a delay as a 'cervical dilatation of less than 2 cm in 4 hours for first labours' and as 'cervical dilatation of less than 2 cm in 4 hours or a slowing in the progress of labour for second or subsequent labours'. These observations should be made once labour has already established and the early labour phase has passed. In other words your cervix has not dilated at this rate but you have been having regular strong surges.

The observation about how dilated your cervix can only be made during a vaginal examination. If you agree to vaginal examinations, your midwife is also going to assess if your baby's head has travelled any deeper into the pelvis and how well the baby's head is applied to your cervix and what the baby's position seems to be at the time of examination. The NICE guideline (2017) requires your midwife to consider all of these observations and interpret these findings as either progress or lack thereof. In the case of a delay your midwife may suggest to you to release your waters.

Releasing the waters will shorten your labour by about an hour and it may increase the strength and pain of your contractions (NICE, 2017). Releasing the waters at this stage may also show the presence of meconium, the baby's first bowel motion. This is important to know because if you are in labour at home or in a midwife led unit, meconium is likely to trigger a transfer to an obstetric hospital. This is because meconium could indicate that your baby is distressed. It could also be entirely benign particularly in a mature baby because babies frequently move their bowels in late pregnancy without there being any problem. It is also important to recognise that releasing the waters can increase your experience of pain and it could take you some time to regulate and get on top of that again either with breathing or with pharmaceuticals.

Whether you agree to having your waters released or not, the guideline states that your midwife is to offer you a further examination after two hours. If there is no progress, your midwife is to transfer your care to the obstetric team who will then discuss your options with you further (NICE, 2017).

Labour augmentation with an oxytocin drip

This is the next step of interventions if your labour was observed as being delayed in the first stage. A synthetic form of the hormone oxytocin will be diluted in saline and given to you in an intravenous drip. The drip gets titrated every half hour until your contractions are 3-4 in every ten minutes. Oxytocin induced contractions are associated with more labour pain and women who receive oxytocin drips in labour describe 'the experience of having their labour augmented as being atypically painful', they considered the augmentation as 'causative of negative childbirth experiences' (Alòs-Pereñígueza, et al., 2023).

You will be offered an epidural prior to starting a drip in order to pre-empt the increase in pain. According to the NICE guidelines (2017), 'using oxytocin after spontaneous or artificial rupture of the membranes will bring forward the time of birth but will not influence the mode of birth or other outcomes'. In other words the baby will be born sooner but when compared to other women who labour without the use of an oxytocin drip in the obstetric unit there is no difference in the rate of caesarean section.

When you interpret this information, bear in mind that this data is all gathered within the system. So just like we have to acknowledge that the data we have about how birth is generally safe for you and your baby, we also have to acknowledge that augmentation does not impact on your mode of birth within this way of approaching labour and birth. There are systems - like the model practised at The Farm - where the intervention rate is significantly lower than that associated with the medical approach to birth (Gaskin, 2007).

Once the oxytocin drip is up and running, the frequency and strength of your contractions will increase. It is also now advised that you have a CTG monitor on because of this increase in strength and frequency of contractions (NICE, 2017).

You'll be advised to have a further vaginal examination 4 hours after starting the oxytocin drip. If your cervix has not opened by at least 2 cm at this examination the need for a caesarean section will be assessed by the medical staff and you will be advised accordingly. If you have progressed, then you will be advised to have further vaginal examinations every 4 hours (NICE, 2017).

Active pushing and the second stage of labour

The second stage of labour is the time between being fully dilated and the birth of your baby.

Ideally you will be in your zone and going with your instinctual urge to push. In the medical model of birth the practice of active pushing is commonly used. Active pushing is what you probably imagine when you think of giving birth to your baby. It is what we see on television and it usually involves a squad of cheerleaders shouting 'push'. It is often used when women have epidurals because when you have an epidural, you won't feel your contractions and you will most likely need direction with your pushes.

Active pushing is also called purple pushing because it involves breath holding. You are asked to take a deep breath, hold your breath, bring your chin to your chest and push into your bottom. The authors of a systematic review concluded that there is no benefit to the practice in women without epidurals and that it is associated with an increased chance of bladder damage (Prins et al., 2011).

In a physiological labour and birth there is no evidence to support the practice of this type of breath holding with your pushes. In my experience women sometimes like some reassurance from the outside and a gentle indication that all is well can be helpful. Women have also asked me to support them with some encouragement if they get very tired. They might want to hear that they are almost there. I encourage you to refer to your sensations often. How could you yourself confirm that your baby is moving? Can you reach down and check? Can you hold your baby as you are shifting your baby down?

If you have an epidural, it's a little different. Once you are fully dilated, usually there's an hour of resting and allowing your body to move the baby down. You might feel some pressure and you might know when to work with your body to move your baby down. You'll learn when to push. If you have no sensations, your midwife will help you by telling you when to push. You can still reach to your baby to get some feedback about how the baby is moving through your birth canal. Sometimes a mirror works well, too, so you can see your baby move with your efforts.

Manual protection of the perineum (MPOP) and episiotomy

An Episiotomy is a surgical incision into your perineal body, performed with sterile scissors. The perineal body is a body of muscle tissue between your vagina and your anus. If it is deemed necessary, it is performed just before the baby's head emerges. Ideally conversations around this will be had before your labour and your consent is gained before an episiotomy is performed.

Episiotomy was first mentioned in obstetric literature in 1742 and by the 1950s it became so embedded in medical childbirth practice that it became a routine intervention . There was a belief that it was protecting the mother and her child and that childbirth without performing an episiotomy was dangerous to the baby and that our perineal muscles could even injure a baby's skull (Cleary-Goldman, 2003). Yes, the underlying presumption was that nature routinely gets it wrong! Thankfully the practice of routine episiotomies at every birth was dropped and NICE guidelines now suggest not to carry them out at a spontaneous vaginal birth (NICE, 2017).

There's evidence that suggests that episiotomies can increase your risk of tearing into your anal sphincter muscle particularly a 'mediolateral' episiotomy. There's also evidence that suggests that an episiotomy that is performed at a 45 to 60 degree angle can have a protective effect for tearing into the sphincter muscle (a third or fourth degree tear). The consensus in the medical community is that if an episiotomy is deemed necessary and you consent to it then it should always be performed at a 45 to 60 degree angle (Cleary-Goldman et al, 2003).

Tearing naturally

As the baby is born, you may have a tear into your soft tissues around the vagina. Any area can be affected, but most commonly it is the perineal body itself. Perineal tears are classified into one of four different categories depending on which part of the soft tissue got damaged.

- A first-degree tear describes a tear into the skin only and if it is not bleeding, your midwife is likely to advise that no repair is needed. Tearing in the skin can happen in the perineal area but also in the labia or near your urethra.

- A second-degree tear involves skin and perineal muscle tissue and your midwife may advise suturing.

- A third-degree tear involves muscle fibres from a circular muscle that controls your back passage, your anal sphincter muscle.

- A fourth-degree tear is a tear that extends into the tissue that forms the separation between your back passage and your vagina, the rectum.

For you as a woman about to give birth it is important to know that third- and fourth-degree tears that are detected and repaired heal well. They affect around 3% of women overall and are more common in a first birth than in a subsequent birth (RCOG, 2015). Third and fourth degree tears are repaired in theatre, usually with a spinal anaesthetic. The recommended aftercare is that you will be prescribed a prophylactic antibiotic to reduce the chance of infection and a laxative so that your stools are soft during your time of healing. You may be referred for physiotherapy and your options for your next birth will be discussed during your next pregnancy (RCOG, 2015).

The OASI Care Bundle

The NICE guidelines recommend that the midwife can either use a 'hands on' or a 'hands off' approach as the baby's head emerges. This means that she either puts her hands on the perineal area and in doing so flexes the baby's head as the baby advances further or watches the perineum with hands off 'but in readiness' (NICE, 2017).

However, this practice is changing since the guideline was issued in 2017 due to the introduction of the OASI care bundle. Between January 2017 and March 2018 a quality improvement project was introduced across the UK after NHS England reported an increase in obstetric anal sphincter injury (OASI) from 1.9% to 5.9% in 2011 (Bitwell, et al., 2021). The quality improvement initiative was first introduced in 16 hospitals in the UK and the evaluation said that the care bundle reduced the overall rate of OASI from 3.3%at the time of introduction of the care bundle to 3%.

The bundle consists of four elements:

- You should be informed about your options around perineal care during your pregnancy

- Your midwife should put a hand onto your perineum during the emergence of your baby's head

- Your midwife or doctor should decide if your perineum is likely to tear badly and do an episiotomy at a 60° angle if they think so

- Staff should recognise and diagnose OASI by use of an examination of the anal sphincter muscle after every birth

(Bitwell, et al., 2021)

The debate about the care bundle

Critics of the bundle have raised concerns that at the point of introduction there was not sufficient evidence to support a widespread use of a 'hands on' approach for every birth. They also questioned whether the increase in reported cases of OASI could be due to an increase in recognition of anal sphincter injury rather than an actual increase in the injury itself (Thornton et al., 2020).

They also point out a study that shows an increase in the rate of episiotomies when a hands on approach was promoted and that a hands on approach didn't reduce the likelihood of injury to your anal sphincter muscle in first time mums whilst increasing the chances of such an injury to mothers of second or subsequent babies. The authors also point out that the implementation of a hands on approach might limit women's choice of birth position and promote lying on your back as a default position again (Thornton, et al., 2020).

The paper I am quoting from here was a critical review of the OASI care bundle written by Jim Thornton and Hanna Dahlen in 2020. The authors also quote an study that showed that perineal warm packs reduced injury to the anal sphincter muscle from 5.8% to 1.9% and that this practice was not included in the care bundle. They also questioned why all women should be subjected to having an examination of their anal sphincter muscle after birth given that this is an unpleasant examination that involves inserting a finger into a woman's back passage in order to assess whether the anal sphincter muscle is intact on palpation. The authors point out that this examination could cause distress and trauma to women, particularly when you have a history of sexual assault (Thornton, et al., 2020).

The authors of the care bundle published a response to similar criticism voiced to them in a letter. In response to the criticism that there was not enough evidence to implement the care bundle the authors said that part of the objective was to produce better quality evidence to guide practice in the future. They stated that in the second part of the quality improvement initiative OASI2 includes a guide for antenatal discussion for practitioners. Discussion about how you would like to approach the care of your perineum as your baby emerges should include, perineal massage, the use of warm compresses, the use of different birth positions and the importance of a slow birth of the baby's head (Thakar, R., et al., 2022).

You can see how complex and complicated every minute aspect of your care can get. For me, as a midwife trying to embrace the big picture here, what stands out is that the reported incidence of sphincter injury by NHS England in 2011 was 5.9% (almost 6 out of every 100 women) and by 2017, when the OASI care bundle was introduced to 16 units in England, the incidence of sphincter injury is reported to be 3.3% (about 7 out of every 200 women). There is variation in the data. The reported reduction in injury is anal sphincter injury withthe OASI care bundle is relatively small. From 33 out of every 1000 women to 30 out of every 1000 women. When talking about their experiences in hindsight, some women feel that a 'hands on' reassured them (Biswell et al., 2021) but women's experiences vary and your preference may be different.

Many of the women I speak to don't think about this part of their birth plan. Women don't know that their midwife may ask them to move into a semi-recumbent position so that the midwife can implement the OASI care bundle which involves assessing for the need of an episiotomy. It is good to be aware during your pregnancy so that you can make an informed choice about your preference. Unless you clearly state your preference, your midwife's practice will most likely be influenced by what they were initially taught, the guidelines in their area of practice and their own preference. Most midwives in the UK prefer a hands-on approach (Stride, et al., 2021).

It also strikes me that the studies and discussions around the OASI care bundle do not consider the potential impact of the birth environment or evaluate the likelihood of injury to the anal sphincter when women birth their babies into their own hands undisturbed and without directed pushing.

So, in summary:

· Your perineum can tear during birth.

· Most tears are uncomplicated and they heal well. Your midwife may advise suturing and suture the tear if you consent.

· There are more complicated tears that involve your anal sphincter muscle, those will usually be repaired in theatre. They take longer to heal and usually you will have physiotherapy after a tear like this.

· These types of tears are more likely in a first birth and the overall incidence hovers around 3%.

· Warm compresses alone can reduce your chance of anal sphincter injury.

· Some hospitals in the UK have implemented the OASI care bundle.

· The care bundle involves assessing the need of an episiotomy and therefore your practitioner may ask you to lie on your back as the baby emerges.

· The OASI care bundle reduces your likelihood of a tear into your anal sphincter muscle by 0.3%.

· The OASI care bundle is not suited for waterbirth, so opting for a waterbirth means opting out of the bundle.

· Some women feel that 'hands on' reassured them, others feel it had a negative effect on their experience of birth.

· You can decline any aspect of the OASI care bundle at birth and you can write your preferences in your birth plan.

How to support healing if you did have a birth injury

· Keep the area clean. Change your pad regularly and use maternity pads. In my experience the sanitary pads that have a plastic type surface can irritate your perineum and cause discomfort and possibly infection (this is my observation, I have never studied this).

· Hydrate – adequate hydration is important for healthy tissue in general, but it also makes your urine less concentrated and reduces stinginess when you pee.

· Nutrition – a healthy, well balanced nutrition is important for overall health in general, but when your body needs support for healing, it is even more important!

· Rest so that your body can heal.

· In the case of infection or a breakdown of the wound, manuka honey preparations can be used to support healing. Ask your midwife if this is the case.

Instrumental birth

An instrumental birth is a birth that involves the use of either a vacuum cup (ventouse) or forceps. In the UK about 1 in 8 mums have an instrumental birth overall. If you are having your first baby, your chances of having an instrumental birth are 1 in 3 (NMPA, 2022; Murphy, et al., 2020).

The most common reason for an instrumental birth is 'prolonged second stage of labour' meaning that the birthing phase (often called the pushing stage) has lasted more than two hours if it is your first baby or more than an hour if you have had a baby before.

Instrumental births are least likely in a midwife led unit (MLU) or at home.

According to the Birthplace Study UK (2011), your risk of an instrumental birth as a first time mum is 126/1000 at home, 118/1000 in a freestanding MLU, 159/1000 in an alongside MLU and 191/1000 in an obstetric led unit. For mums who have had babies before, the risk is 9/1000 at home, 12/1000 in a freestanding MLU, 23/1000 in an alongside MLU and 38/1000 in an obstetric led unit. These figures show that the risk is significantly lower once you have had a baby before. They also show that your risk is highest in an obstetric led unit and this is reflective of the fact that epidurals are associated with an increased chance of having an instrumental birth and upright positions and staying up on your feet moving freely are common practices in the MLU and at home.

If you are in a midwife led environment, a transfer to obstetric led care will be initiated if your birthing phase is by the above definitions prolonged and if it doesn't look like the birth of your baby is imminent within the next hour. This protocol is based on the NICE guidelines for intrapartum care (2017) in the UK which states that the birth of the baby should be expected within three hours of active second stage for first time mums and two hours for second time mums.

The rationale to limit the birthing stage is that during this stage babies' blood oxygen supplies become depleted at a faster rate than they do in the first stage of labour. Because of this, it is generally suggested that if you wish to get more time to give birth to your baby without the use of an instrument, a CTG monitor should be applied and your baby's heart rate should be observed more closely so that an instrumental birth can be performed if it looks like your baby is getting stressed (NICE, 2017).

Which instrument is recommended depends on your baby's position in the pelvis. I often get asked if you can opt for a caesarean section instead of an instrumental birth and this is a more complex topic because if the head is deep in the pelvis, a caesarean can be the more complicated procedure. Generally there is time to discuss your options with your midwife and doctor even at this late stage in labour (RCOG, 2020). The only reason there may not be time to discuss is if your baby appears to be stressed and the birth needs to be speeded up.

There are some risks attached to an instrumental birth. You are very likely to have an episiotomy and your risk of having a 3rd or 4th degree tear is increased. It occurs in up to 4 in 100 women following a ventouse and between 8 and 12 women in every 100 women following a forceps birth. You are also at an increased risk of bleeding heavily after an assisted birth. Your baby can have bruises or cuts on the head from the instrument itself. This happens in about 1 in 10 babies. Bruising increases your baby's risk of jaundice (5-15 in 100 babies) and 5-15 out of every 10 000 babies experience bleeding on the brain because of an instrumental birth (RCOG, 2020).

Have conversations with your care providers early. Ask at different facilities what their instrumental birth rates are so that you can choose a place where this is least common.

Ways to minimise your risk of having an instrumental birth include choosing a midwife led environment, staying active and upright in labour and having the continuous support from someone you know in labour in addition to your care provider. This could be your partner or a doula. Avoiding an epidural or, if you opt for one, lying on your side can also decrease your chances of having an instrumental birth (RCOG, 2020).

About the length of second stage

I already mentioned that a delay in the second stage of labour is one of the common indications for an instrumental birth. So what is considered a delay?

Dr. Friedman (1955) defined the normal maximum length of the second stage of a first labour as 2.5 hours. The NICE guidelines (2017) reflect this. They state that birth in most first time mothers should occur after three hours of an active second stage of labour and that a delay in the second stage should be diagnosed after two hours of active second stage. The active second stage is defined as follows: the baby's head is visible, expulsive contractions (an urge to push) combined with a finding of a fully dilated cervix on vaginal examination or other signs of a fully dilated cervix; findings of a fully dilated cervix and directed pushing in the absence of an urge to push. When routine vaginal examinations are performed, there is the possibility that you are found to be fully dilated but you don't feel any urge to push. Consider that the clock on your second stage of labour starts once you are fully dilated. This is something to consider when you think about whether or not you would like vaginal examinations.

Whilst the evidence base for initially introducing this time limit on the second stage of labour is arguably poor, it is also important to note that there are some disadvantages the longer the pushing stage lasts. In a literature review of four studies with participants ranging between 78 and 103 415 women Newman (2017) found that spontaneous vaginal birth rates increase with a longer pushing time therefore negating the risks of caesarean section for some women, but there are also small increases in morbidities for mum and baby associated with extended second stages. Those included slight increases in 3rd and 4th degree tears and infection in the newborn baby. The author concluded that the effect on the baby was 'negligible'. A further study on the length of the second stage concluded that there were no ill effects on babies with prolonged second stages but that mothers were more likely to bleed heavily after the birth, have a 3rd or 4th degree tear and infection after the birth (Matta, et al., 2019).

This is another complex topic and for you, the main question really is how you can be proactive around avoiding an instrumental birth. For your birth plan, consider where you will have your baby, how you want your progress to be monitored, how do you feel about the time frames in labour in general and in the second stage particularly, what about movement in labour? What are your plans around pain relief?

Listen to the Midwives' Cauldron episode 'Pushing and Cervixes' for a great exploration of this very topic. Sign up to the extra resources page to find a quick link to it.

Caesarean birth

Caesarean sections can happen in labour or they can be planned. Any caesarean birth that happens in labour is called an unplanned caesarean birth or sometimes an emergency caesarean section. Approximately 1 in 5 women overall have an unplanned caesarean birth. If you are having your first baby the likelihood increases to around 1 in 3 women who start out in labour (RCOG, 2022).

Unplanned caesarean births are categorised by the degree of urgency.

A Category 1 Caesarean birth happens when there is an immediate threat to your or your baby's life. Your baby will be born as soon as possible and within 30 minutes. This could be because of an emergency situation such as a drop in your baby's heart rate that does not resolve.

A Category 2. Caesarean birth happens when you or your baby are showing signs of distress but the situation is not immediately life-threatening. In this case your baby will be born within 75 minutes. This could be because of a delay in the second stage of labour when you and baby are both fine.

A Category 3. Caesarean section is when there is no immediate problem but the baby needs to be born. This could be because of a delay in the first stage of labour when there are no concerns about you or your baby..

A Category 4. Caesarean Birth is timed to suit you or your healthcare provider. This is a planned caesarean birth or sometimes an elective caesarean section.

(NICE, 2021)

Here's what happens at a caesarean section:

- An anaesthetist speaks to you about your pain relief options - usually you will be able to stay awake

- You will have urinary catheter sited

- You will have a shave of your pubic area

- You will have two intravenous cannulas for fluids

- You will be offered prophylactic antibiotics to be given before the incision of your skin, these are to help prevent infections like UTI and wound infections in your recovery time

- You will have bloods taken and sent off

- Your leg will be measured for compression stockings and those will be put on

- You will change into a theatre gown

- Your partner will be given a gown or scrubs to slip on for when they join you in theatre

- You will be wheeled into theatre directly or into an anaesthetic room

- Your spinal anaesthetic will be administered - in category 1 situation, this may be a general anaesthetic

- You will be draped and your partner can join (if you didn't have a general anaesthetic)

- Once your anaesthetic is effective, the operations can start

- Antibiotics are given

- An incision will be made along your bikini line, the surgeon works in layers to get to your womb

- Your baby will be lifted out and to you which can take a few minutes, sometimes forceps are needed to lift the baby out of your pelvis

- Your baby can go skin to skin with you right away and you can still delay cutting the cord

- Your partner can cut the cord if you ask for this before the section

- The anaesthetist will give an oxytocin drug to contract the womb so the placenta separates

- The placenta is removed

- Your womb and muscles are sutured, the skin can be sutured or closed with clips

- You and your baby will go to a recovery area where you will be monitored for about an hour. You will be helped with feeding your baby

Things you can ask for:

- Have the dots to monitor your heart be stuck to the edge of the chest so your baby doesn't lie on them during skin to skin

- Have your cannula placed into the non-dominant arm or hand

- Have the sats probe on a finger on your non-dominant arm

- Your birth music to be played

- The screen to be lowered so you see your baby emerge

- Assist with lifting your baby onto your own chest

- Partner to cut the cord

- Low voices so your (and your partner's) voice is the first thing the baby hears

- For baby to stay skin to skin the whole time in theatre and to be transferred with the baby skin to skin

These are possible in non urgent or semi urgent caesareans. In a category 1 situation the priority will shift to getting the baby born and clinicians will do their best to keep you informed whilst performing all the procedures mentioned above. You may need a general anaesthetic in a category 1 situation because giving you a spinal would take too long. If you are asleep for the operation, your birth partner will be asked to wait in a separate room. The midwives will usually bring your baby to them and they can have skin to skin whilst they wait for you to wake up. In those cases you will usually get a full explanation of what happened and why it all happened after the event. You can also ask for a conversation with the doctor who was with you at the time.

Active versus physiological management of the third stage of labour (birth of the baby's placenta)

Your baby's birth is complete only when the placenta is born. Your baby's placenta is expelled when your womb contracts some time after the birth of your baby. When you leave this up to nature, this happens spontaneously. In maternity care this is called physiological management and it is to a degree defined by the omission of a drug that makes your womb contract. When you have that drug, this is called active management.

When you seek routine maternity care, there are protocols and time frames for both of those scenarios regardless of your birth setting. So let's look at active versus physiological management of the third stage of labour as defined by the NICE Intrapartum care guidelines (2017).

Physiological management	Active management
No injection is given	Injection of a drug called oxytocin into your thigh, usually as you give birth
The cord is clamped and cut once it has stopped pulsing	The cord is clamped and cut between 1 and 5 minutes after the birth
You push the placenta out If this doesn't happen within an hour of the birth of your baby, a delay in third stage of labour is diagnosed	The placenta is pulled out by the midwife once there are signs that it has separated from the wall of the uterus (womb) A delay is diagnosed if this doesn't happen within 30 minutes of the birth of your baby

Whether you choose one or the other is a personal decision and what you choose will depend on your values, your general health, your pregnancy health and it will likely depend on your previous birth experiences.

When the placenta separates, there is an initial blood loss and that is absolutely normal, your body has the reserves for this and you normally have a bleed of up to half a litre or 500 ml at the birth of the placenta. When your blood loss exceeds 500 ml, we call this a minor postpartum haemorrhage and when it exceeds 1000 ml and you develop symptoms associated with rapid and excessive blood loss, it's classed as a major haemorrhage (Begley CM, et al., 2019). Not being able to stop such a bleed would be very dangerous and it can be fatal. There is a range of drugs that we have at hand in order to help if someone bleeds more than normal after the birth of the baby but when the bleeding doesn't stop that way, you will be brought to theatre. There are various surgical interventions that can stop the bleeding and the last line of treatment would be to remove your womb. You will see the overall likelihood of bleeding discussed below.

In order to minimise the chances of excessive bleeding after birth, the NICE intrapartum guidelines suggest that every woman in the UK is **advised** to have active management regardless of risk factors. The guideline further suggests that those women who have no risk factors and request physiological management should be supported in it (NICE, 2017).

What the NICE guidelines say about physiological management:

- About 5 in 100 women will suffer nausea and vomiting

- Approximately 29 out of 1000 women will have a postpartum bleed of more than 1 litre of blood

- About 40 in 1000 women will have a blood transfusion following the birth of their baby

What the NICE guidelines say about active management:

- It shortens the time between your baby being born and the placenta being expelled

- About 10 in 100 women will suffer nausea and vomiting

- About 13 in 1000 women will have a postpartum bleed of more than 1 litre of blood

- About 14 in 1000 women will have a blood transfusion after birth

These statistics reflect all women giving birth regardless of risk factors. A Cochrane review from 2019 concluded that it was unclear if there was any advantage of active management for women with no risk factors for postpartum haemorrhage (Bekeley, et al, 2019). Having said that, I think that birth physiology cannot purely be defined by omitting a medicine. Smooth physiological placental birth without a haemorrhage requires a surge of oxytocin in the mother and no time frames. It should be preceded by a physiological birth of the baby. It is also paramount that the room is warm, quiet and that there is no sense of anxiety or any coming and going of strangers. Mother and baby should not be separated at this stage and they should be free to interact at the mother's pace (Reed, 2022). In modern maternity care in the UK, after an hour of waiting a physiological third stage of labour is considered to be prolonged and interventions will be suggested. Dr Rachel Reed suggests that true birth physiology rarely unfolds in the industrial obstetric model, even if the birth is described as a 'spontaneous vaginal birth' and that therefore a case could be made for advising active management for most women. She states that 'Active management of the placenta will reduce the chance of a PPH in a setting that does not support physiology and in which routine intervention is the norm. [...] Physiological placental birth is an option, and possible if you manage to avoid induction, augmentation, an epidural or complications – but be aware of how difficult it may be, and don't beat yourself up if it doesn't happen' (Reed, 2022).

Routine practices to be aware of in the context of the birth of the placenta:

If you would like a physiological third stage and would like to wait for longer than an hour, you will need to point this out to your providers in advance of labour. Third stage of labour is still labour and in its physiology it favours quiet and calm. You need to be able to interact with your baby, and ideally your baby will crawl to your breast and latch for a first breast feed. For this to happen naturally, disturbances should be kept to a minimum. There should not be any palpation of your womb and your baby should be left on with you with the cord attached.

Weighing your baby, getting armbands applied, and putting a hat on your baby should wait until the placenta is born.

Hat or no hat?

If you are giving birth in a birth centre or hospital, you may be offered a hat for your baby immediately after the birth. This is because babies lose heat via their damp little heads and their temperature can drop quickly. A body temperature below 36.5 °C is called hypothermia. Hypothermia is a challenge for babies and can lead to serious problems such as difficulty maintaining normal blood sugar levels, poor feeding, and a slowing down of the breathing rate. In severe cases of hypothermia a baby may need hospital admission to a neonatal unit. Babies more at risk of becoming too cold include premature babies, babies who are growth restricted or babies whose blood sugars are low but all babies are considered to be at risk of hypothermia within the first 12 hours of life (Waldron, et al., 2007). A warm environment, drying the baby after birth and immediate skin to skin with a mum whose temperature is normal can help prevent hypothermia (Vilinski, et al., 2014). As well as immediate skin to skin, parents are also often offered a hat for their newborn baby to reduce heat loss from the head and reduce the risk of hypothermia.

Disadvantages of putting a hat on a baby immediately at birth include that you can't smell your baby's head. Smelling your baby's body odour has been associated with changes in the brain that contributed to bonding (Lundström, et al., 2013). In my experience, a hat can also take your focus away from interacting with your baby or disrupt breastfeeding if it falls off and gets put on again a lot.

If you would like your baby to wear a hat immediately after birth, it may be worth bringing a cotton bonnet that you can tie on in order to prevent it from falling off a lot. If you would like not to have a hat on your baby immediately after the birth you will need to state it clearly in your birth plan.

Deciding if you would like Vitamin K for your baby

Every parent is offered an injection of Vitamin K for their baby at birth. Vitamin K can also be given as oral drops. I often meet parents who have never heard about it at all and when they are either in labour or have just had a baby, it is difficult to give a truly informed overview of what the injection is for.

In short, vitamin K helps your baby's blood clotting in case they have an internal bleed that we don't know about. Here's some more information for informed decision making:

The condition we are trying to prevent by giving your baby Vitamin K is:

HDN - Haemorrhagic Disease of the Newborn also called
VKDB - Vitamin K Deficiency Bleed

For the purpose of this overview I am going to use the term HDN because it doesn't imply an innate deficiency every human has at birth but rather an occasional disease process that we can help or try to prevent with vitamin K.

It is impossible to predict who will develop HDN.

A baby with HDN may have bleeding, get pale, be fussy, vomit, not be interested in feeding or be very lethargic and sleepy and will need to go to the intensive care unit. The baby can experience complications like a bleed on the brain and a baby can die from HDN or sustain brain damage. So the problem is potentially very serious.

Trying to determine the absolute risk of a baby getting HDN when they are not given vitamin K is difficult. There was no randomised controlled trial (RCT) before routine prophylaxis was introduced. In the absence of an RCT we have to rely on literature from before vitamin K was introduced. The average incidence of Vitamin K deficiency bleeding in high income countries is about 1/11000 babies who didn't receive Vitamin K at birth

(Wickham, 2017). Dr Sara Wickham discusses the variations in numbers and the problems when trying to establish a true reflection of what the incidence would be without routinely giving Vitamin K in great detail in her book 'Vitamin K and the Newborn' and I highly recommend reading it (Wickham, 2017).

If vitamin K is given by intramuscular injection at birth or soon after, the incidence of HDN is estimated to drop to 1/100000 (from an average of 1/11000 in high income countries). The preparation that is most commonly used is called Konakion MM.

We don't have numbers as specific for oral vitamin K and again, I refer you to Dr Wickham's book to read about the considerations around oral vitamin K. We do know that it offers some protection and that it is important to know that it needs to be given with a feed for better absorption.

The disadvantages to giving vitamin K by injection are related to the dangers in relation to giving an injectable drug. Very rarely a wrong drug can be given, if that happens it could be drugs that would have been intended for mums. I personally know of a friend's niece who received a drug intended for her mother. The baby was very ill and had to go to intensive care as a result. There are further anecdotal stories of babies receiving pethidine (a pain relief drug commonly used in labour) or Syntometrine (a drug commonly used for the birth of the placenta) (Wickham, 2017). Either of those can be very dangerous for a baby. Those are isolated cases, there are no statistics for them because this happens so rarely.

Other injection specific disadvantages are that it's sore and there is possibility for infection at the injection site (BNF, 2022).

Dangers of the drug itself are difficult to ascertain because it would take a very large study to ascertain possible serious side effects.

The general consensus among the medical community is that the perceived and measured benefits of vitamin K injections at birth in relation to preventing the serious and potentially fatal condition of HDN outweigh any potential serious side effects.

The decision of whether you want your baby to have vitamin K is yours, it's okay to decline. For a very detailed and nuanced discussion about what to consider when you decide to decline, give oral vitamin K or give vitamin K by injection, please read Dr Wickham's book, it is the most comprehensive discussion on the subject I have ever read.

Important note:

Regardless of your decision, a baby who is lethargic, doesn't feed, pee or poo or who is displaying any concerning symptoms at all needs an urgent medical review. Always mention if you have declined Vitamin K in such a circumstance even if not asked.

Conclusion

Thank you so much for reading my first book.

I sincerely hope that you found value in the pages and I wish you all the best on your birth journey.

Your pregnancy and birth education doesn't have to stop here! Would you like to have some in person support from me? I offer one to one pregnancy coaching sessions where you can ask me questions directly and get clear on what's important to you before you have your baby.

Would you like to get to know other parents on the same journey as you? You can get on your R.O.A.D. To Birth via zoom. Preparing alongside others is fun and it often forms bonds that last for a lifetime.

Join the R.O.A.D. To Birth community today:

Don't forget to download your Bonus Materials at https://www. essentiallybirth.com/sevensecretsbonuspage

My favourite books about pregnancy, birth and life in general (in alphabetical order)

Beverly Engel - The Nice Girl Syndrome: Stop Being Manipulated and Abused - and Start Standing Up for Yourself

David R. Hawkins - Letting Go: The Pathway of Surrender

Dr Sarah Buckley - Gentle Birth, Gentle Mothering: A Doctor's Guide to Natural Childbirth and Gentle Early Parenting

Dr Sara Wickham - Group B Strep Explained

Dr Sara Wickham - In Your Own Time: How western medicine controls the start of labour and why this needs to stop

Dr Sara Wickham - Inducing Labour: making informed decisions

Dr Sara Wickham - Vitamin K and the Newborn

Dr Rachel Reed - Reclaiming Childbirth as a Rite of Passage: Weaving Ancient Wisdom with Modern Knowledge

Ina May Gaskin - Spiritual Midwifery

Janet Balaskas - New Active Birth: A Concise Guide to Natural Childbirth

Jenny Blyth - The Down to Earth Birth Book: a practical guide to natural birth

Kerstin Uvnas-Moberg - The Oxytocin Factor: Tapping the Hormone of Calm, Love and Healing

Sarah Schmid - Freebirth - Self-Directed Pregnancy and Birth

References

Corbett, G. A., et al., (2022). Onset and outcomes of spontaneous labour in low risk nulliparous women. European Journal of Obstetrics & Gynecology and Reproductive Biology, 274, 142–147.

NICE (2021). Inducing labour. NICE guideline [NG207]. Accessed via: https://www.nice.org.uk/guidance/ng207

Pistollato, F. et al (2015) ,Plant-Based and Plant-Rich Diet Patterns during Gestation: Beneficial Effects and Possible Shortcomings, American Society for Nutrition. Advanced Nutrition 2015;6:581–91. Accessed via: https://www.ncbi.nlm.nih.gov/pmc/articles/PMC4561836/

Wickham, S. (2021). In Your Own Time: how western medicine controls the start of labour and why this needs to stop. Avebury: Birthmoon Creations.

SANDS Charity Link: https://www.sands.org.uk/

About risk and risk factors:

MBRRACE-UK: Mothers and Babies: Reducing Risk through Audits and Confidential Enquiries across the UK (2014) Definitions of terms used in the MBRRACE-UK Perinatal Mortality Surveillance Report.

https://www.npeu.ox.ac.uk/assets/downloads/mbrrace-uk/reports/MBRRACE-UK-PMS-Report-2014-Definitions-of-terms.pdf

MBRRACE-UK: Mothers and Babies: Reducing Risk through Audits and Confidential Enquiries across the UK (2019). Saving Lives, Improving Mothers' Care. Lessons learned to inform maternity care from the UK and Ireland Confidential Enquiries into Maternal Deaths

and Morbidity 2017-19 https://www.npeu.ox.ac.uk/assets/downloads/mbrrace-uk/reports/maternal-report-2021/MBRRACE-UK_Maternal_Report_2021_-_FINAL_-_WEB_VERSION.pdf

MBRRACE-UK: Mothers and Babies: Reducing Risk through Audits and Confidential Enquiries across the UK (2021) Key Messages from the report 2021 Infographic.

https://www.npeu.ox.ac.uk/assets/downloads/mbrrace-uk/reports/maternal-report-2021/MBRRACE-UK_Maternal_Report_2021_-__Infographic_v10.pdf

MBRRACE-UK: Mothers and Babies: Reducing Risk through Audits and Confidential Enquiries across the UK (2021) Perinatal Mortality Surveillance Report. UK Perinatal Deaths for Births from January to December 2019

https://www.npeu.ox.ac.uk/assets/downloads/mbrrace-uk/reports/perinatal-surveillance-report-2019/MBRRACE-UK_Perinatal_Surveillance_Report_2019_-_Final_v2.pdf

Nursing & Midwifery Council (2019). Standards of proficiency for midwives. Retrieved from https://www.nmc.org.uk/globalassets/sitedocuments/standards/standards-of-proficiency-for-midwives.pdf

Royal College of Obstetricians and Gynaecologists (2013). Induction of labour at term in older mothers (Scientific Impact Paper No. 34). London: RCOG.

https://www.rcog.org.uk/media/lp4n13jn/sip_34.pdf

Dr. Sara Wickham (2021). In Your Own Time: how western medicine controls the start of labour and why this needs to stop. Avebury: Birthmoon Creations.

Are you at increased risk of developing a blood clot:

Jacobson B, et al. (2019). Safety and Efficacy of Enoxaparin in Pregnancy: A Systematic Review and Meta-Analysis. Advances in Therapy. 2020;37(1):27-40.

NIH (2022). Enoxaparin. National Library of Medicines. National Center for Biotechnology Information. Last update 10 September 2022. Accessed on 20th September, 2022 via https://www.ncbi.nlm.nih.gov/books/NBK539865/

Royal College of Obstetricians and Gynaecologists (2015). Reducing the Risk of Venous Thromboembolism during Pregnancy and the Puerperium Green-top Guideline No. 37a. London: RCOG. Accessed via https://www.rcog.org.uk/media/qejfhcaj/gtg-37a.pdf

Are you at increased risk of developing high blood pressure or pre-eclampsia:

American College of Obstetricians and Gynecologists (2018). ACOG committe opinion. Number 743. Committee on Obstetric Practice. Society for Maternal–Fetal Medicine. Low-dose aspirin use during pregnancy. Accessed via https://www.acog.org/clinical/clinical-guidance/committee-opinion/articles/2018/07/low-dose-aspirin-use-during-pregnancy

Hastie, et al. (2021). Aspirin use during pregnancy and the risk of bleeding complications: a Swedish population-based cohort study. American Journal of Obstetrics and Gynecology. Volume 224, Issue 1, P95.E1-95.E12. Accessed via https://www.ajog.org/article/S0002-9378(20)30737-7/fulltext

Joint Formulary Committee (2022) 'Aspirin', in British National Formulary. Accessed via: https://bnf.nice.org.uk/drugs/aspirin/

National Health Service (2021). Side effects of low-dose aspirin. Accessed via: https://www.nhs.uk/medicines/low-dose-aspirin/side-effects-of-low-dose-aspirin/

National Institute for Health and Care Excellence. Hypertension in pregnancy: quality standard . Manchester (United Kingdom): NICE;

2013. Accessed via: https://www.nice.org.uk/guidance/qs35/resources/hypertension-in-pregnancy-2098607923141

Pistollato, F. et al (2015) ,Plant-Based and Plant-Rich Diet Patterns during Gestation: Beneficial Effects and Possible Shortcomings, American Society for Nutrition. Advanced Nutrition 2015;6:581–91. Accessed via: https://www.ncbi.nlm.nih.gov/pmc/articles/PMC4561836/

Rolnik, et al. (2017). Aspirin versus Placebo in Pregnancies at High Risk for Preterm Preeclampsia. The New England Journal of Medicine. 377: 613-622 Accessed via: https://pubmed.ncbi.nlm.nih.gov/28657417/

Royal College of Obstetricians and Gynaecologists (2022). Information for you. Pre-Eclampsia. London: RCOG. Accessed via: https://www.rcog.org.uk/media/rnulgc5d/pi_pre-eclampsia-2022.pdf

Are you at an increased risk of developing diabetes in pregnancy:

Gestational Diabetes UK (2022). Accessed via: https://www.gestationaldiabetes.co.uk/diagnosing-gestational-diabetes/

Hegerty, C.K. (2020), The new gestational diabetes: Treatment, evidence and consent. Australian and New Zealand Journal of Obstetrics and Gynaecology, 60: 482-485. Accessed via: https://doi.org/10.1111/ajo.13116

Royal College of Obstetricians and Gynaecologists (2012). Shoulder Dystocia. Green–top Guideline No. 42. 2nd Edition

Hansen, et al. (2014). Shoulder dystocia: Definitions and incidence. Seminars in Perinatology. Volume 38, Issue 4, Pages A1-A4, 183-234

Are you at an increased risk of developing anaemia in pregnancy:

Dr Miriam Martinez-Biarge (2022). Plant-based diets for pregnancy. Lecture. University of Winchester. Attended as part of the Plant-based nutrition; a sustainable diet for optimal health course in June 2022

Joint Formulary Committee (2022) 'Ferrous Fumerate', in British National Formulary. Available at: https://bnf.nice.org.uk/drugs/ferrous-fumarate/

Pavord, et al. (2020). UK guidelines on the management of iron deficiency in pregnancy. BJ Haem. Volume 118. Issue 6. Pages. 819-830

Royal College of Obstetricians and Gynaecologists (2015). Blood Transfusion in Obstetrics Green-top Guideline No. 47. Accessed via: https://rcog.org.uk/media/sdqcorsf/gtg-47.pdf

Is your baby at risk of being growth restricted/SFH measurement and growth charts:

Gardosi J, et al. (2013). Maternal and fetal risk factors for stillbirth: population based study. British Medical Journal. 346:f108. Accessed via: https://www.bmj.com/content/346/bmj.f108.long

Hugh, O., Williams, M., Turner, S. and Gardosi, J. (2021), Reduction of stillbirths in England from 2008 to 2017 according to uptake of the Growth Assessment Protocol: 10-year population-based cohort study. Ultrasound Obstet Gynecol, 57: 401-408. Accessed via: https://obgyn.onlinelibrary.wiley.com/doi/epdf/10.1002/uog.22187

NHS England (2019). Saving Babies' Lives v.2 Care Bundle

https://www.england.nhs.uk/wp-content/uploads/2019/03/Saving-Babies-Lives-Care-Bundle-Version-Two-Updated-Final-Version.pdf

Perinatal Institute for Maternal And Child Health (2020). Growth Assessment Protocol Guidance (GAP) Accessed via: https://perinatal.org.uk/GAPguidance.pdf

RCOG (2014). The Investigation and Management of the Small–for–Gestational–Age Fetus.

Green–top Guideline No. 31. Accessed via: https://www.rcog.org.uk/media/t3lmjhnl/gtg_31.pdf

UK stillbirth trends in over 11 million births provide no evidence to support effectiveness of Growth Assessment Protocol program - GAP

https://obgyn.onlinelibrary.wiley.com/doi/10.1002/uog.21999

Have you had a caesarean section before:

Royal College of Obstetricians and Gynaecologists (2015). Birth after Previous Caesarean Birth (Green-top Guideline No. 45). Accessed via: https://www.rcog.org.uk/guidance/browse-all-guidance/green-top-guidelines/birth-after-previous-caesarean-birth-green-top-guideline-no-45/

Royal College of Obstetricians and Gynaecologists (2016). Information for you. Birth options after previous caesarean section. Accessed via: https://www.rcog.org.uk/media/na3nigfb/pi-birth-options-after-previous-caesarean-section.pdf

Urine screening and the other blood tests:

Dr. Sara Wickham (2019). Group B Strep explained. 2nd edition. Birthmoon Creations

Public Health England (2019). SMI B41: UK Standards for Microbiology 640 Investigations-Investigation of urine. United Kingdom Accessed via: https://www.gov.uk/government/publications/smi-b-41-investigation-of-urine

Royal College of Obstetricians and Gynaecologists (2017). Prevention of Early-onset Group B Streptococcal Disease (Green-top Guideline No. 36). Accessed via: https://www.rcog.org.uk/guidance/browse-all-guidance/green-top-guidelines/prevention-of-early-onset-group-b-streptococcal-disease-green-top-guideline-no-36/

Are you rhesus negative:

Bio Products Laboratory Limited (2022). D-Gam. Accessed via: https://www.medicines.org.uk/emc/product/9724/smpc

CSL Behring (2021). Rhophylac. Accessed via: https://www.drugs.com/pro/rhophylac.html

Dr Sara Wickham (2021). Anti-D Explained. Birthmoon Creations

National Institute for Health and Care Excellence (2008). Routine antenatal anti-D

prophylaxis for women who are rhesus D negative. NICE. Accessed via: https://www.nice.org.uk/guidance/ta156/resources/routine-antenatal-antid-prophylaxis-for-women-who-are-rhesus-d-negative-pdf-82598318102725

Qureshi, H., et al. (2014), BCSH guideline for the use of anti-D immunoglobulin for the prevention of haemolytic disease of the fetus and newborn. Transfusion Med, 24: 8-20. Accessed via: https://doi.org/10.1111/tme.12091

On ultrasound scans in general:

Beech, B.; Robinson, J. (1994). Ultrasound? Unsound. AIMS. Accessed via:

https://www.aims.org.uk/assets/media/26/ultrasound-unsound.pdf

BMUS (2009). Guidelines for the safe use of diagnostic ultrasound equipment. Prepared by the Safety Group of the British Medical Ultrasound Society. Accessed via: https://www.bmus.org/static/uploads/resources/BMUS-Safety-Guidelines-2009-revision-FINAL-Nov-2009.pdf

Choosing a place of birth:

Brocklehurst, et al. (2011). Perinatal and maternal outcomes by planned place of birth for healthy women with low risk pregnancies: the Birthplace in England national prospective cohort study. BMJ (British Medical Journal), 343, d7400. Accessed via: https://www.npeu.ox.ac.uk/birthplace#the-birthplace-cohort-study

Guidelines and Audit Implementation Network (2018). Guideline for admission to midwife-led units in Northern Ireland. Normal labour & birth pathway. RQIA. Accessed via: https://www.rqia.org.uk/RQIA/files/3a/3a7a37bb-d601-4daf-a902-6b60e5fa58c2.pdf

Hutton, et al. (2019). Perinatal or neonatal mortality among women who intend at the onset of labour to give birth at home compared to women of low obstetrical risk who intend to give birth in hospital: A systematic review and meta-analyses. EClinicalMedicine. 2019;14:59-70. Published 2019 Jul 25. doi:10.1016/j.eclinm.2019.07.005 Accessed via: https://pubmed.ncbi.nlm.nih.gov/31709403/

Reitsma, et al. (2019). Perinatal or neonatal mortality among women who intend at the onset of labour to give birth at home compared to women of low obstetrical risk who intend to give birth in hospital: A systematic review and meta-analyses. EClinicalMedicine, 2019. Accessed via:

https://www.thelancet.com/journals/eclinm/article/PIIS2589-5370(20)30063-8/fulltext

Freebirth

Association for the Improvement of Maternity Services Website: https://www.aims.org.uk/information/item/freebirth

Birth Trauma Association Website (2018). What is birth trauma. Accessed via: https://www.birthtraumaassociation.org.uk/for-parents/what-is-birth-trauma

Birthrights. Unassisted Birth. Accessed via: https://www.birthrights.org.uk/factsheets/unassisted-birth/

Dahlen (2020). Birthing Outside the System: The Canary in the Coal Mine. Routledge Research in Nursing and Midwifery

Gloucestershire Hospitals NHS Foundation Trust. Maternity Information for those considering giving birth unassisted by a midwife. Accessed via:

https://www.gloshospitals.nhs.uk/media/documents/Unassisted_birth_leaflet_FINAL_110521_1.pdf

Renfrew et al (2014) Midwifery and quality care: findings from a new evidence-informed framework for maternal and newborn care. The Lancet, vol 384, no 9948, pp 1129-1145 https://www.ncbi.nlm.nih.gov/pubmed/24965816

Royal College of Midwives (2019). RCM Clinical Briefing Sheet: 'freebirth' or 'unassisted childbirth' during the COVID-19 pandemic. Accessed via:

https://www.rcm.org.uk/media/3923/freebirth_draft_30-april-v2.pdf

Sarah Schmid (2015). Freebirth - Self-Directed Pregnancy and Birth: Basic knowledge | Illustrations and photos | Personal stories. Edition Riedenburg E.U.; 1st edition

WHO (2019) Maternal mortality. Accessed via: https://www.who.int/en/news-room/fact-sheets/detail/maternal-mortality

Membrane Sweeps

Finucane EM, Murphy DJ, Biesty LM, Gyte GML, Cotter AM, Ryan EM, Boulvain M, Devane D. Membrane sweeping for induction of labour. Cochrane Database of Systematic Reviews 2020. Accessed via: https://www.cochrane.org/CD000451/PREG_membrane-sweeping-induction-labour

National Institute for Health and Care Excellence (2021). Inducing labour. Accessed via: https://www.nice.org.uk/guidance/ng207

If your waters release before labour

National Institute for Health and Care Excellence (2017). Intrapartum care for healthy women and babies. Accessed via: https://www.nice.org.uk/guidance/cg190

National Institute for Health and Care Excellence (2021). Inducing labour. Accessed via: https://www.nice.org.uk/guidance/ng207

Dr. Sara Wickham (2021). In Your Own Time: how western medicine controls the start of labour and why this needs to stop. Avebury: Birthmoon Creations.

Induction of Labour

Dahlen, et al (2021). Intrapartum interventions and outcomes for women and children following induction of labour at term in uncomplicated pregnancies: a 16-year population-based linked data study. BMJ Open. 2021;11(6):e047040. Accessed via: https://pubmed.ncbi.nlm.nih.gov/34059509/

Joint Formulary Committee (2022) 'Dinoprostone', in British National Formulary. Available at: https://bnf.nice.org.uk/drugs/dinoprostone/ (Accessed: 21 August 2022).

Middleton P, et al. (2018). Induction of labour for improving birth outcomes for women at or beyond term. Cochrane Database of Systematic Reviews. Accessed via: https://www.cochranelibrary.com/cdsr/doi/10.1002/14651858.CD004945.pub4/full

Middleton P, et al. (2020) Induction of labour at or beyond 37 weeks' gestation. Cochrane Database of Systematic Reviews 2020, Issue 7. Art. No.: CD004945. Accessed 04 November 2022 via: https://www. cochranelibrary.com/cdsr/doi/10.1002/14651858.CD004945.pub5/full

Dr. Sara Wickham (2021). In Your Own Time: how western medicine controls the start of labour and why this needs to stop. Avebury: Birthmoon Creations.

Early Labour

Rolnik, et al. (2017). Aspirin versus Placebo in Pregnancies at High Risk for Preterm Preeclampsia. The New England Journal of Medicine. 377: 613-622 Accessed via: https://pubmed.ncbi.nlm.nih.gov/28657417/

The Undercover Midwife (2015). Paracetamol in labour. Blog post. Accessed via: https://undercovermidwife.blogspot.com/2015/03/paracetamol-and-labour.html

Routine observations in labour

Moncrieff G, et al. (2022). Routine vaginal examinations compared to other methods for assessing progress of labour to improve outcomes for women and babies at term. Cochrane Database of Systematic Reviews 2022, Issue 3. Art. No.: CD010088. DOI: 10.1002/14651858.CD010088.pub3.

National Institute for Health and Care Excellence (2017). Intrapartum care for healthy women and babies. Accessed via: https://www.nice.org.uk/guidance/cg190

CTG Monitoring

Alfirevic, Z., et al (2017). Continuous cardiotocography (CTG) as a form of electronic fetal monitoring (EFM) for fetal assessment during labour. Cochrane Database of Systematic Reviews 2017, Issue 2. Art. No.: CD006066. DOI: 10.1002/14651858.CD006066.pub3. Accessed 02 October 2022

National Institute for Health and Care Excellence (2017). Intrapartum care for healthy women and babies. Accessed via: https://www.nice.org.uk/guidance/cg190

Small, K.A. et al., (2020). Intrapartum cardiotocograph monitoring and perinatal outcomes for women at risk: Literature review. Women and Birth. Volume 33, issue 5, pp. 411-418. Accessed via: https://pubmed.ncbi.nlm.nih.gov/31668871/

Small, K.A. et al., (2022). The social organisation of decision-making about intrapartum fetal monitoring: An Institutional Ethnography. Women and Birth. Available online 18 September 2022. Accessed via: https://www.sciencedirect.com/science/article/abs/pii/S1871519222003225

How labour progress is monitored

Gaskin IM. (2002),Spiritual Midwifery. 4th edn. Summertown, TN: Book Publishing Company

NMPA Project team (2022). National Maternity and Perinatal Audit: Clinical Report. Based on births in NHS maternity services in England and Walesbetween 1 April 2018 and 31 March 2019. Accessed via: https://www.hqip.org.uk/wp-content/uploads/2022/06/Ref.-336-NMPA-annual-report-FINAL.pdf

Pain Relief in Labour:

Bohren MA, et al., (2017). Continuous support for women during childbirth. Cochrane Database of Systematic Reviews. Accessed via: https://www.cochranelibrary.com/cdsr/doi/10.1002/14651858.CD003766.pub6/full

Cluett ER, Burns E., (2018). Immersion in water in labour and birth. Cochrane Database Systematic Review. Accessed via: https://pubmed-ncbi-nlm-nih-gov.hsclib-ezp.qub.ac.uk/29768662/

Jones L, et al. (2012). Pain management for women in labour: an overview of systematic reviews. Cochrane Database of Systematic Reviews. Accessed via: https://www.cochranelibrary.com/cdsr/doi/10.1002/14651858.CD009234.pub2/full

Lawrence A, et al., (2013). Maternal positions and mobility during first stage labour. Cochrane Database of Systematic Reviews. Accessed via: https://www.cochranelibrary.com/cdsr/doi/10.1002/14651858.CD003934.pub3/full

Rodriguez, M.A. (2005). Pain Mechanisms: A New Theory: A gate control system modulates sensory input from the skin before it evokes pain perception and response. British Journal of Midwifery, 13(8): 522-526

RCOA (2019). Risks associated with your anaesthetic. Section 10: Headache after a spinal or epidural injection. Accessed via: https://www.rcoa.ac.uk/sites/default/files/documents/2022-06/10-HeadachesSpinalEpidural2019web.pdf

RCOA (2020). Epidural pain relief after surgery. Accessed via: https://www.rcoa.ac.uk/sites/default/files/documents/2022-06/05-EpiduralPainRelief2020web.pdf

Weibel S, et al., (2017). Patient controlled analgesia with remifentanil versus alternative parenteral methods for pain management in labour.

Cochrane Database of Systematic Reviews. Accessed via: https://www. cochranelibrary.com/cdsr/doi/10.1002/14651858.CD011989.pub2/full

Artificial rupture of membranes

National Institute for Health and Care Excellence (2017). Intrapartum care for healthy women and babies. Accessed via: https://www.nice.org.uk/ guidance/cg190

Labour augmentation

Alòs-Pereñíguez, S., et al., (2023). Women's views and experiences of augmentation of labour with synthetic oxytocin infusion: A qualitative evidence synthesis. Midwifery, Volume 116, 2023. Accessed online November 5th, 2022 via: https://www-sciencedirect-com.hsclib-ezp.qub. ac.uk/science/article/pii/S0266613822002637?via%3Dihub

Gaskin IM. (2002),Spiritual Midwifery. 4th edn. Summertown, TN: Book Publishing Company

National Institute for Health and Care Excellence (2017). Intrapartum care for healthy women and babies. Accessed via: https://www.nice.org.uk/ guidance/cg190

Active pushing

Prins M, et al., (2011). Effect of spontaneous pushing versus Valsalva pushing in the second stage of labour on mother and fetus: a systematic review of randomised trials. BJOG 2011;118:662–670.

MPOP and Episiotomy

Ayuk, P. et al. (2019). Obstetric anal sphincter injuries before and after the introduction of the Episcissors-60: a multi-centre time series analysis. Eur. J. Obstet. Gynecol. Reprod. Biol., 241 (2019), pp. 94-98

Bidwell, P. et al. (2021). Women's experiences of the OASI Care Bundle; a package of care to reduce severe perineal trauma. Int Urogynecol J 32, 1807–1816. https://doi.org/10.1007/s00192-020-04653-2

Cleary-Goldman, J., & Robinson, J. N. (2003). The role of episiotomy in current obstetric practice. Seminars in Perinatology, 27(1), 3–12

RCOG (2015). The Management of Third- and Fourth-Degree Perineal Tears. Green-top guideline no. 29. Accessed via: https://www.rcog.org.uk/media/5jeb5hzu/gtg-29.pdf

Stride, S., et al. (2021).Identifying the factors that influence midwives' perineal practice at the time of birth in the United Kingdom. Midwifery. November 2021

Thakar, R., et al. (2022). Authors' reply re: OASI Care Bundle. BJOG: Int J Obstet Gy, 129: 175-176. https://doi-org.hsclib-ezp.qub.ac.uk/10.1111/1471-0528.16901

Thornton, J.G., Dahlen, H.G. (2020). The UK Obstetric Anal Sphincter Injury (OASI) Care Bundle: A critical review, Midwifery, Volume 90, 102801, ISSN 0266-6138, https://doi.org/10.1016/j.midw.2020.102801.

Instrumental Birth

Friedman EA. (1955). Primigravid labor: A graphicostatistical analysis. Journal of the American Academy of Obstetrics and Gynecology; 6:567–89

Matta, P., et all., (2019). Prolonged second stage of labour increases maternal morbidity but not neonatal morbidity. Aust N Z J Obstet Gynaecol, 59: 555-560. https://doi-org.hsclib-ezp.qub.ac.uk/10.1111/ajo.12935

Murphy, DJ, et al. (2020), on behalf of the Royal College of Obstetricians Gynaecologists. Assisted Vaginal Birth. BJOG 2020; 127: e70– e112.

Newman M. (2017). Does extending time limits in the second stage of labour compromise maternal and neonatal outcomes? British Journal of Midwifery. 2017;25(8):506-510.

NMPA Project team (2022). National Maternity and Perinatal Audit: Clinical Report. Based on births in NHS maternity services in England and Walesbetween 1 April 2018 and 31 March 2019. Accessed via: https://www.hqip.org.uk/wp-content/uploads/2022/06/Ref.-336-NMPA-annual-report-FINAL.pdf

RCOG (2020). Information for you. Assisted vaginal birth (ventouse

or forceps. Accessed via: https://www.rcog.org.uk/media/2p4fh2kd/pi-vaginal-birth-final-28042020.pdf

Caesarean Birth

RCOG (2022). Information for you. Considering a caesarean birth. Accessed via:

https://www.rcog.org.uk/media/41jdfprf/considering-a-caesarean-birth-patient-information-leaflet.pdf

RCOG (2022). Planned Caesarean Birth. Consent Advice No. 14. Accessed via: https://rcog.org.uk/media/33cnfvs0/planned-caesarean-birth-consent-advice-no-14.pdf

NICE (2021). Caesarean birth. NICE guideline [NG192]. Accessed via: https://www.nice.org.uk/guidance/ng192/chapter/Recommendations#factors-affecting-the-likelihood-of-emergency-caesarean-birth-during-intrapartum-care

Active versus physiological management of the third stage of labour

Begley CM, et al. (2019). Active versus expectant management for women in the third stage of labour. Cochrane Database of Systematic Reviews 2019, Issue 2. Accessed via:

https://www.cochranelibrary.com/cdsr/doi/10.1002/14651858.CD007412.pub5/full

Mavrides E, et al. (2016) on behalf of the Royal College of Obstetricians and Gynaecologists. Prevention and management of postpartum haemorrhage.BJOG 2016;124:e106–e149. Accessed via: https://www.rcog.org.uk/guidance/browse-all-guidance/green-top-guidelines/prevention-and-management-of-postpartum-haemorrhage-green-top-guideline-no-52/

National Institute for Health and Care Excellence (2017). Intrapartum care for healthy women and babies. Accessed via: https://www.nice.org.uk/guidance/cg190

Reed, R. (2022). Midwife thinking blog. An actively managed placenta may be the best option for most women. Accessed via: https://midwifethinking.com/2015/03/11/an-actively-managed-placental-birth-might-be-the-best-option-for-most-women/

Hat or no hat?

Lundström, J., et al. (2013). Maternal status regulates cortical responses to the body odor of newborns. Frontiers in Psychology. Volume 4. Accessed via: https://www.frontiersin.org/articles/10.3389/fpsyg.2013.00597/full#h7

Vilinski, et al., (2013). Hypothermia in the newborn: An exploration of its cause, effect and prevention. British Journal of Midwifery. Volume

22 · Issue 8. Accessed via: https://www.britishjournalofmidwifery.com/content/clinical-practice/hypothermia-in-the-newborn-an-exploration-of-its-cause-effect-and-prevention

Waldron, S. et al., (2007). Neonatal thermoregulation. Infant. volume 3. issue 3. Pp. 101-104. Accessed via: https://www.infantjournal.co.uk/pdf/inf_015_nor.pdf

Deciding if you would like Vitamin K for your baby

Joint Formulary Committee (2022) 'Phytomenadione', in British National Formulary. Available at: https://bnf.nice.org.uk/drugs/phytomenadione/

Dr Sara Wickham (2017). Vitamin K and the Newborn. Birthmoon Creations

Printed in Great Britain
by Amazon

22737328R00142